GERMS, BIOLOGICAL WARFARE, VACCINATIONS

Germs, Biological Warfare, Vaccinations

WHAT YOU NEED TO KNOW

Gary Null, Ph.D.

with James Feast

SEVEN STORIES PRESS

NEW YORK

A Seven Stories Press First Edition

Seven Stories Press
140 Watts Street
New York, NY 10013
http://www.sevenstories.com

In Canada: Hushion House, 36 Northline Road, Toronto, Ontario M4B 3E2

In the U.K.: Turnaround Publisher Services Ltd., Unit 3, Olympia Trading Estate, Coburg Road, Wood Green, London N22 6TZ

In Australia: Palgrave Macmillan, 627 Chapel Street, South Yarra VIC 3141

Library of Congress Cataloging-in-Publication Data

Null, Gary.
    Germs, biological warfare, vaccinations : what you need to know / Gary Null, with James Feast.—1st ed.
        p. cm.
    Includes bibliographical references.
        ISBN 1-58322-518-8 (pbk.)
    1. Bioterrorism. 2. Communicable diseases—Prevention. 3. Communicable diseases—Alternative treatment. 4. Vaccination—Complications 5. Alternative medicine. I. Feast, James. II. Title.

RC88.9.T47 N855 2002
616.9'045—dc21
2002151606

9 8 7 6 5 4 3 2

College professors may order examination copies of Seven Stories Press titles for a free six-month trial period. To order, visit www.sevenstories.com/textbook, or fax on school letterhead to (212) 226-1411.

Book design by Cindy LaBreacht

Printed in Canada

Contents

Preface

---

*On ne peut faire une bonne physionomie qu'en accordant
toutes nos contrariétés, et il ne suffit pas de suivre une suite
de qualités accordantes sans accorder les contraires.* [You
can only produce a good portrait by harmonizing all our
contrary qualities, and it is not enough to trace a series of
harmonious qualities without harmonizing their opposites.]

—Blaise Pascal, *Pensées*

Two incidents can be taken as exemplums of disturbing disease trends that
will only become more prominent as the twenty-first century unfolds.

The first involves tuberculosis (TB) in New York City. In the nineteenth
century, tuberculosis was a scourge that felled millions and sent others to
mountain sanitariums for drawn-out and costly treatments. However, once
the proper antibiotics were identified, TB was driven back until, by the middle of the twentieth century, it was nearly forgotten in the West and, when it
did occur, easily extinguished.

But, later in the century, the disease gained a second wind. In New York
State, "after 1975 it [tuberculosis] began a slow resurgence, with the number
of TB reports rising like a rocket from 1980 to 1989."[1] The increase testified to
a number of minuses in American medicine. Inferior healthcare for the poor
was one problem, what with the large number of uninsured having to rely on
emergency room care or go without treatment. Couple that with overcrowd-
ing and constantly deteriorating conditions in the prisons, where most of the

transmission of the disease was occurring. Add to that a weak public health system, which, since the election of Reagan in 1980, had been shortchanged at the federal level by Republican presidents. However, all these things going wrong did not touch the most frightening aspect of the whole situation, which was due to nature's adaptive powers. Many tuberculosis cases in this resurgence were of a new variant of the illness. "One strain, dubbed 'W,' was resistant to so many drugs that it was essentially untreatable."[2]

Eventually, under the firm hand of New York City Commissioner of Health Dr. Margaret Hamburg, this mini-epidemic would be quelled. However, two disquieting facts about the problem remain. It would take at least six weeks for labs to determine which drug combinations could knock out this new strain—and it wasn't the only new TB form that cropped up. Moreover, this disease was an immigrant. W "had originated in Russia in the final years of the Soviet Union. And as early as 1988 fully a quarter of all New York City TB cases had been among foreign-born individuals."[3] The importation of this disease was promoted by the increasing globalization of air travel between nations combined with the decreasing United States funding for monitoring the health of those entering the country and taking care of them once here. President Carter had created an Office of Refugee Health "to screen incoming immigrants for a host of communicable diseases and to serve as a cultural bridge for their entry into the mainstream medical system."[4] Under Reagan's tenure, this office was defunded and more or less ceased functioning.

The second exemplary incident occurred in 1971 in Aralsk, a town in Kazakhstan in what was then the Soviet Union. It concerned an outbreak of smallpox. This second disease, whose kill rate was once greater than that of tuberculosis, did away with 500 million people in the twentieth century, more than went down in all the wars of the period. As with TB, drugs and medical treatment eventually put this disease to rest. In 1967 the World Health Organization (WHO) set out to eliminate the disease, and by 1977 could rightfully say that smallpox was gone from the earth.

However, the small outbreak in 1971 is significant not because it is one of the last, but because of its peculiar etiology. Only now is the full story becoming known. In June 2002, a team of experts from the Monterey Institute of International Studies made public a report that was the first to give details of what happened.

Aralsk is on the coast of the Aral Sea, sitting downwind of Vozrozhdeniye Island, which during the Cold War was the Soviet Union's major test site for biological weapons. A United States parallel might be Arizona and New

Mexico, which were the preferred proving grounds for United States nuclear detonations.

As the *New York Times* summarizes the Monterey Institute study, "A ship doing ecological research sailed too close to a military smallpox test that sent out a deadly plume, infecting a crew member who carried the virus back to the city."[5] In Aralsk, two children and a young woman died from the disease, and many were taken sick, including seven who had already been vaccinated. The government rushed to quell the budding epidemic. "Nearly 50,000 residents of Aralsk were vaccinated in less than two weeks, and hundreds were placed in isolation in a makeshift facility on the edge of town.... Travel to and from Aralsk was stopped, and many homes were disinfected."[6]

This report comes at a bad time for the Bush administration, which has been pushing for a mass smallpox vaccination to guard the citizenry against terrorist threats. The Monterey group said, given the smallpox strain released by the Russians was so potent that it downed even those who had been vaccinated, this "raises questions about whether new vaccines or drugs might be needed if this strain were used in an attack."[7] In other words, what's the use of mass vaccinations if they are carried out with vaccines to which laboratory-developed pathogens are impervious?

The Monterey study caused the Bush administration to take notice. In a role reversal, D.A. Henderson, a top bioterrorism expert who counsels the secretary of Health and Human Services, downplayed the findings. Normally, experts like Henderson get busy magnifying the danger of terrorism, giving their own field more importance; but, in this case, the expert dismissed the shocking implications, expressing skepticism about the report's conclusions. Henderson stated, "We don't know when they [the Soviets who caught the illness] were vaccinated or whether they were successfully vaccinated," and added that the reports' authors were "jumping to far-reaching conclusions with scant information."[8]

The fact remains that such examples of germs "improved" in bioterrorist laboratories throw into doubt the value of vaccines and other drug-based methods of defense. As we will see in detail, those creating bioweapons are well aware of and consistently create countermeasures against any prophylactic means that would derail their plans of spreading illness.

And there is a second depressing thought conveyed by this episode. Assuming smallpox was indeed released accidentally during a biological warfare exercise—the government still denies this incident took place—it could just as well have occurred in 1981, after the elimination of smallpox, as in 1971, since the Soviets went on experimenting with weaponizing smallpox through the 1980s. There will never be any escape from mankind's scourges as long as biological weapons are created and, as recent experience showed, willingly or unwittingly used.

(We might add that although the government has never officially admitted that this smallpox outbreak was due to weapons testing, the Russian government did confess to a similar incident. In May 1992, Boris Yeltsin, president of Russia, admitted that, in 1979, there was a leakage of anthrax spores from a military laboratory in Sverdlovsk. As a paper reported, because of this release, "an estimated one thousand people…eventually died from anthrax, a disease that without treatment is usually fatal in two weeks.… [Once aware of the accident] the Soviet military seized control of the area, covering the contaminated ground with fresh topsoil."[9])

Introduction

THE APPEARANCE OF MORE DANGEROUS GERMS

In Laurie Garrett's monumental and magisterial *Betrayal of Trust: The Collapse of Global Health*, two themes are brought together that *should not be but are* constantly separated in discussions of current disease issues. These are the interlocking problems for our health posed by the *natural* and *humanly engineered* growth of new diseases. Bioterrorism experts whose books have been commanding the marketplace of late, given the 2001 mailborne anthrax attacks, understandably disregard the topic of the growth of prophylactic-resistant germs that are occurring naturally due to germs' adaptive capacities. Nonetheless, beyond the obvious fact that these are all new health threats, which present unexpected challenges to a medical system oriented toward the alleviation of individual health problems, not large-scale disease outbreaks, there are three broad ways in which these two types of illness are closely linked.

1. The viruses or bacteria that produce these diseases, whether they appear through human intervention or by way of natural evolution, will be hardier than previous generations. Bioterrorists select the most powerful, treatment-resistant form of a given disease for their campaigns. Moreover, those who have the funding to engage in more scientifically driven biological warfare, as did the Soviet Union, whose massive, well funded, and well-stocked Biopreparat Research Institute was engaged in high-level development of biological weapons for decades, can bioengineer germs that combine the most reprehensible qualities of more than one disease producer.

The first hard evidence of the creation of stronger microbes, by the way, came in the 1998 publication in a British scientific journal of an article by Russians who had worked for Biopreparat. In the paper, they detailed how they had inserted genes from a harmless bacteria into anthrax, producing a new entity that could resist penicillin and vaccines and was able to enter right into cells, something natural anthrax could not do. Nobelist Joshua Lederberg commented, on seeing this paper, "This, as far as I know, is the first example of an artificially contrived pathogen."[1]

Meanwhile, naturally occurring germ mutations, fueled by mismanaged healthcare, are proving stronger than the antibiotics that once summarily dealt with them.

Medical care plays a part in creating these super-bugs in a number of ways. On one hand, for example, where illness is treated haphazardly, as in the former Soviet Union, more resistant germs are cultivated. There the fall of Communism led quickly to widespread breakdown of the medical delivery system. Since drugs were unobtainable from doctors or hospitals, people would rely on places like the Deserters Bazaar in a major city in Georgia, where "quacks and marketers...bolstered the...misuse of antibiotics," which they would prescribe with all the confidence of ignorance.[2]

The only foolproof way to conquer an antibiotic-eliminable disease is to carry on the assault using *one* effective drug until all traces of the disease causer are gone. Depending on such an erratic supply sources as "street pharmacists," which involved the buyer in a constant switch between antibiotic types, meant that before a germ was eliminated by one drug, the ailing person had switched to another, which gave the germ a chance to successfully mutate to a more resolute form.

On the other hand, to take a second problem, in the United States, due to the disappearance of epidemics, there has been a relaxation of stringent control laws over carriers of contagious diseases. So, in the aforementioned New York TB outbreak, resistant TB strains were created, not by capricious use of antibiotics, but because of premature breaking off of the normal round of treatment. Garrett describes the situation by taking as an illustration Harlem hospital where in 1989, 88 percent of TB patients "disappeared before being cured. The patients stopped their antibiotics as soon as they felt better, but before the bacteria was completely gone from their systems, thus allowing drug-resistant tuberculosis strains to emerge."[3]

This same author presents a litany of other ways the world's anarchic, largely underfunded medical facilities have been contributing to the birth of superbugs. These include "sloppy infection control practices in hospitals," the overuse of antibiotics, which are often "misprescribed, and, in nearly half of all common infections, prescribed to treat viral [which they can't affect] rather than bacterial infections."[4] She also notes that a fear of being sued for not doing enough pushes physicians to prescribe the most powerful, across-the-board antibiotics where simpler ones would do. Moreover, the widespread feeding of antibiotics to livestock, where they are useful as fattening agents not as disease preventers, means bacteria can often develop resistance in the souped-up animals, and then pass into human circulation through poorly cooked meat or eggs. In fact, European nations, recognizing this danger, ban the use of antibiotics in animal feed; but the United States' greedy farmers and pharmaceutical manufacturers have stopped such prohibitions from making it into law. Remember, today the bulk of antibiotics are sold in America not to alleviate human stresses but as additives to animals' feed.

Thus our first point is that, whether through the diabolic ingenuity of terrorist scientists or defaults in the world's medical culture, a new wave of engineered or evolutionarily improved bugs is being created and will be unleashed on our society.

---

2. A second connection between bioweapons and naturally occurring enhanced germs is that when they appear they will face United States healthcare institutions incapable of handling them.

For one, since many of the diseases that are likely to be used by bioterrorists, such as smallpox, are ones that haven't been seen for decades, doctors will not be sure how to handle them or even recognize them. The latter problem was highlighted in February 1999 when Dr. John Bartlett, by way of an experiment, went into Johns Hopkins University hospital and asked for advice about an (imaginary) patient who had all the symptoms of inhalational anthrax infection. The doctor who was asked his opinion said the patient had the flu. Then Bartlett went to the radiology department with an X-ray of a person infected with inhalational anthrax. Again, the symptoms were misdiagnosed. He proceeded through the hospital, never getting the correct diagnosis. He later published his findings, showing that none of the doctors he consulted had a clue to the real nature of the disease that was being described to them. As the authors of *Living Terrors* make clear,

"Bartlett wasn't trying to say that his city was less prepared for disaster than other cities…his point was that signals could be missed anywhere."[5]

Once one of these hardy diseases appears and its correct nature is deciphered, it is unlikely we will be able to fight it off in a timely manner. For one, our national immunization programs, though still active, have been underfunded so that in many regions they have become shells of their former selves. Furthermore, those alienated from medicine, whether because, like many poor minorities in urban settings, they have been cut out of the healthcare loop, or because, like many libertarians in the West, they feel immunization is a government intrusion on their rights, have kept their children from being vaccinated.

(Later, though, we will question whether immunization is really as valuable as it is cracked up to be. What we are getting at in the following paragraphs is not the crying need for vaccinations of all types. Rather we are simply underscoring that government programs in the field of children's healthcare are hardly carried out with the diligence necessary.)

Garrett argues that the danger of lower child vaccination rates was made clear in a measles epidemic that hit the United States from 1989 to 1991. Over 55,000 children came down with the disease. As she sees it, the easy spread of measles was helped by the incomplete vaccination of poor children. In New York City, for instance, 20 percent of children on Medicaid were without the shots.

> Drastic cuts in federal support for health care programs for the poor, coupled with the Medicaid block grant shift to the states, meant that fewer children in New York City even saw doctors…[and these children] were less likely…to get properly vaccinated against measles or other child killers.[6]

On top of this, the production of vaccines or specialized antibiotics to deal with diseases that haven't been seen recently or ones such as anthrax, that occur very occasionally, has been allowed to lapse, so that stocks are not available in case of sudden spikes in disease occurrence.

Behind all this, as the quote on measles makes clear, is a contraction of government spending on public health. This is rationalized by doctrines of individualist conservatism, which are promulgated by New Right think tanks, given bowdlerized presentation in the mainstream media, and adopted in a popularized form by many of the public. According to this position, the government should stop funding social programs and creating cushions for those left out by the market economy. Rather this economy should be let alone to regulate itself, so that people sink or swim depending on their own luck or pluck. "No more free lunches and no life preservers" is the conservatives' cry.

This is disingenuous on two fronts. The wealthy individuals and corporations who are funding the crusade are not so much interested in downsizing government as a spur to individualism, but as a way to further reduce taxes. Moreover, the most important leaders elected under the new battle cry of "Less government" have applied their vision selectively, slashing away at healthcare and welfare programs, while concurrently beefing up military budgets, agribusiness subsidies and various corporate welfare schemes.

Most notoriously President Ronald "Chopping Block" Reagan, came to power promising to rein in the spendthrift ways of the federal bureaucracy. At his inauguration, he promised, "It is my intention to curb the size and influence of the federal establishment."[7] A month later he laid out his plans to accomplish this curbing by reducing spending and eliminating the nation's budget deficit. But, as Garrett points out, "In his two terms of office, Reagan would actually increase federal government spending, eclipsing the one trillion dollar mark, largely through rising military expenditures."[8]

All this spelled trouble for public health, which was not among conservatives' favored programs. After all, the very *raison d'être* of public health is collective health, while the conservatives see healthcare as an individual matter.

We need to explain public health's mission more directly. This system is centrally concerned with epidemic disease, which it seeks to prevent by insuring a community has pure water, proper sanitation, fresh foods, clean air, and other contributors to a wholesome environment. If an epidemic does begin, public health is in the business of the quick recognition, diagnosis and tracking of the outbreaks, and their speedy containment through quarantines, mass inoculations, and other community-broad efforts.

Such collectively oriented efforts don't sit well with New Right ideologues. They are so far gone on their free market pipe dreams that, for example, in 1988 the premier New Right think tank, the Heritage Foundation, actually argued democracy's public health system should be sold to the highest bidder. The foundation presented a report that "called for privatization of many public health activities, and levying of fees, rather than taxes, to cover the cost of such things as water safety testing."[9] Dr. Michael Osterholm, Minnesota State Epidemiologist, commented acerbically, "How could the public ever feel safe… if its food, water, health care infrastructure, air, schoolchild health…

were handled by private companies that had no accountability, needed to make profits off the process, and possibly had conflicts of interest?"[10]

3.This leads us to a third and final congruence between bioterrorist-delivered and naturally recalcitrant germs. **Since either form, upon its appearance, would profit from gaping holes in our public health structure as well as from the low level of health in the general populace, a rational response to the threat they pose would be correspondent responses: a refurbishment of our neglected public health system to make it ready to hold in check outbreaks of new disease and an improvement in our general health to make those struck in an epidemic likely to survive.** Most of our book will turn on the last-named component and will be taken up with explaining how an individual can improve his or her health radically, although the first point will constantly be kept in mind.

BRIEF EXCURSUS ON THE NATURE

OF THE HUMAN BEING

Two Emphases in Personality and Medicine

———

Here we come to one of the subthemes of the book. It might be said that the two strategies just mentioned are at loggerheads. After all, you might say, doesn't an obsessive concern with taking care of one's own health, through detoxification, vegetarianism, lifestyle modification and so on, point in the very direction of narcissistically individualist medicine that a moment ago was censured as driving the public away from a realistic concern for public health? That would be certainly seem to be a reasonable question.

However, we will argue that two layers in a single human personality structure are at issue here: an egoist and a collectivist level. As our argument develops, we will have to call out some heavy guns, in the form of the founders of sociology, to indicate the philosophical grounding of this view.

However, at this point, we will merely say, that both personality emphases can be found in different medical disciplines, and these emphases can be sorted according to whether they belong to the traditional or newly emerging paradigm. (More about how to characterize those paradigms in a minute.)

Traditional medicine (as seen in virology, for instance) takes its role to be the beating back of illness, which will be accomplished by identifying and striking down a disease agent. This ties in with egoist (or Lockean) individualism insofar as it views people's activities as essentially that of identifying and pursuing goals. Contrawise, alternative medicine (which appears in

such fields as immunology and public health) looks at disease as a disturbance across a number of continuums. While the disease breakdown is most
evident in the affected single human, it is causally related to the meshwork
that links that human to his or her social group and to that group's fuller
community. This ties in with our idea of the collectively oriented (or Mea-
dian) individual whose actions are viewed not solely as the product of un-
trammeled free will, but as part and parcel of the framework of decisions
that have been made by social groups and wider society. [Note: a fuller ex-
planation of this discrepancy between virology and immunology is found in
AIDS: A Second Opinion.[11]

The notion we want to develop is *not* that society is formed of two types
of people: avaricious, conspicuously consuming yuppies (Lockean individualists) and saintly, Gaia-conscious New Agers (Meadean individualists).
Rather, we argue each person contains two strains of individuality. Philosophies and religions have, each in their own way, recognized this. Christianity, for example, has seen humans pulled between earth and heaven. To take
a typical expression of this doctrine, from a thinker we will discuss more
fully in a moment, we may draw from Pascal.

> Signs of the greatness and misery of man are so patent that
> true religion must necessarily inform us both that there is
> some great root of greatness in man [*quelque grand
> principe de grandeur en l'homme*], and also a great root of
> misery. Further it must account for these amazing contra-
> dictions."[12]

In the Christian tradition, humans started out endowed with divine levels of knowledge, health, and understanding, but their rebellion against
their Maker introduced a spiritual pollution that corrupted intelligence,
health, and inter-human sympathy. Pascal puts it like this, "We are composed of two natures, opposite and different in kind, viz. body and soul."[13]
Our fall drove a wedge into our natures. "This double nature [*Cette duplicité*]
in man is so obvious that there are some who thought we have two souls."[14]
In mixed despair and hope, Pascal calls out, "What a monster then is man.
[*Quelle chimère est-ce donc que l'homme!*] Universal judge and helpless
worm…glory and off-scouring of the universe."[15]

In Christianity, the intense split in humanity is correlated to the presence of intertwined divine and animal natures. Nothing is said about collective sentiments. However, if we turn to a foundational work in the field of

sociology, *The Division of Labor in Society* by Emile Durkheim, we see a persuasive statement that the religious ethos is created as a way to depict the collective nature of society. He uses the nature of punishment to illustrate this.

> When we demand the repression of crime it is not because we are seeking a personal vengeance, but rather vengeance for something sacred which we vaguely feel is more or less outside and above us. Depending upon time and place, we conceive this object in different ways.... Very often we represent it to ourselves in the form of one or several concrete beings: ancestors or a divinity.... These sentiments, *because of their collective origin*...stand radically apart from the rest of our consciousness.... Since these sentiments are collective, it is not us that they represent in us, but society.[16]

For Durkheim, a sense of being a part of society is both inescapable and hard to grasp. So while throughout history people have vaguely understood that their lives were deeply molded and inflected by being part of a human group, they have usually not directly voiced this feeling but embodied it in beliefs about ruling gods and fates. For him, the much-discussed difference between human's spiritual and material yearnings represents, at bottom, a veiled depiction of the uneasy dialogue present in everyone between group- and self-oriented projects and aspirations.

Properly, the discussion of this interrelation of personality factors will only play a small role here, acting more as a background notation than a conspicuous theme. Two other deeper positionings, one related to public health, one related to paradigm shifts, will also play such subsidiary, grounding parts. I will refer to them briefly before setting out the agenda of this book.

BIOTERRORISM AND PUBLIC HEALTH

Probably the greatest scandal in the government's preparations for a response to biological terror is how, just as in the budget prioritization we outlined above, the military has been getting the lion's share of monies while public health remains in the cold. Whatever rationale such a division of spoils may have in relation to other types of terrorist attacks, this is unconscionable in relation to biological warfare, where almost all major steps, from identifying what pathogen is in use, to treating casualties, and preventing the spread of the epidemic (in the case of a contagious disease) would be in the hands of public health agencies.

Ignoring this simple truth, law enforcement has been made the centerpiece of biological warfare (BW) preparation. Garrett reports that from 1997 to 1999 "the FBI had the lead role in training local firefighters...in first response to biological attacks."[17] Moreover, the aforementioned Michael Osterholm, Minnesota government epidemiologist and respected expert on biological warfare, notes the same skewed allocations in Clinton's year 2000 anti-terrorism budget. Out of $10 billion overall, only $1.4 billion went to biological and chemical warfare, and of that public health got a sliver, $41 million. The author compares the public health numbers to money spent the previous year on training the national guard ($52 million), buying protective gear for cities ($69.5 million), and training firefighters ($80 million). After assessing these and other law enforcement-related expenses, Osterholm trenchantly concludes, "Most of these funded projects will have *no impact* on our ability to respond to a bioterrorism event."[18] Then, turning analytic, he notes, "Priorities…seem to be determined more by which federal agencies are best at budgetary brinkmanship that by where the money might do the most good."[19]

The wrongheadedness of this approach can be seen in Garrett's description of what went on in April 1996 in Washington, D.C., when FBI and police personnel were faced with an attack on B'nai B'rith headquarters with letters containing (what seemed to be) plague and anthrax. (This turned out to be a hoax.) Although the law-enforcement agencies have never acknowledged any mistakes in their procedures, health experts have pointed out: (1) they isolated only the mailroom, when the air conditioning would have already spread the germs to the whole building; (2) they used chlorine as the one decontaminant to kill the bugs, while most biologists see anthrax as resistant to chlorine; and (3) they took employees outside and sprayed them with fire hoses, which would have "spread the organisms into an aerosolized mist that could rain over the area."[20]

This should make clear that giving a disproportionate amount of money to criminal justice agencies to prepare for bioterrorist assaults is absurd and counterproductive. And there is a even bigger issue in the wings: our government's inappropriate militarization of solutions to problems that will not respond to such treatment.

After the World Trade Center attack, there were mounting fears among liberals that the Bush administration would use the real terrorist threat as an excuse to push through draconian laws that went beyond what was necessary, thereby encroaching on civil liberties. Valid as such fears might be, an equally important point about the dangers of the administration's actions was not pressed. Sending in the army to batter Afghanistan or other states said to harbor terrorism as a *primary* action is as flawed as trying to prepare for BW by pouring money into justice departments.

Again, this is not the appropriate forum for long-winded political discussions, but we will at least be able to suggest that public health can play a role not only in coping with terrorist-sponsored disease outbreaks, but even in forestalling bioterrorists before they strike.

Perhaps surprisingly, this theme will not be pursued by tracing the history of public health measures down through the centuries. Rather, we will concentrate on a single incidents when dramatic changes in the government were made as the only way of coping with an epidemic. This occurred in the 1793 yellow fever outbreak in Philadelphia. We will show how only a progressive, radical democratization of the political functioning allowed the city to stand firm against the disease.

PASCAL IN AN ERA OF PARADIGM SHIFT

Mais les parties du monde ont toutes un tel rapport et un tel enchaisenement l'une avec l'autre, que je croys impossible de connositre l'une sans l'autre et sans le toute. [But the parts of the world are in such correspondence and are so tied together the one with the other that I believe it is impossible to know any one without knowing the other and the whole.]

—Blaise Pascal, *Pensées*

The last subtheme we will cover is that of paradigm shift. Blaise Pascal, whose life straddled such a shift in the most dramatic fashion, will provide our point of departure.

First some background. With some simplifying, we can say that Pascal was one of the two or three greatest thinkers of the seventeenth century. He didn't found merely one science, but seemed to create new branches of mathematics and physics like a flint throwing off sparks. These new branches included hydrology, hydrostatics, and infinitesimal calculus.

As did Francis Bacon, Pascal saw experiment as the royal road to scientific discovery. Let's use his experiments with mercury as an example. Since then-accepted Aristotelian theory (backed by Catholic Church doctrine) argued that vacuums could not exist, the theory was hard put to explain the following simple events. A long glass tube was filled with mercury, then, with a finger covering the open end, it was immersed in a pan of mercury.

The finger removed, the mercury descended a certain depth. Experimenters asked: Was the empty space at the top of the tube a vacuum?

Doctrinaire anti-vacuumists, such as the leading philosopher René Descartes, came up with fantastic explanations, such as: an especially refined, subtle air, slithered between the mercury beads and got in the upper tube. But for those who believed a vacuum could exist, and did so at the top of the tube, there was still the question of what made the mercury drop down only a certain distance. Why wasn't the liquid metal, according to gravity, forced to empty the tube altogether? What caused the mercury to remain at a certain elevation?

Pascal theorized it was air pressure, that is, the weight of the air pressing down against the mercury in the bowl that partially counterbalanced gravity and held the mercury in the tube aloft. He, then, came up with an ingenious experiment to prove this. He had a friend do the mercury experiment in the small town of Clermont, then carry the apparatus to the top of the nearby Puy du Dôme Mountain. It turned out the mercury was lower up on the mountain, indicating that at that high altitude the air pressure was less. This was to be expected since mountain air is thinner in that less air is above it, pressing down. Pascal had both proven the existence of a vacuum and of atmospheric pressure.

By 1654, when Pascal was just thirty-one, he had established himself as a leading light of European science. Although a conventional Christian, he was also a man of the world, going to parties, gaming, meeting fellow intellectuals for talk and argument. Then on November 23, 1654, he was struck by a thunderbolt: a mystical visitation from God that caused him to change his whole life.

He recorded what happened on that fateful evening on a slip of paper which was only discovered after his death. He hid the paper in his clothes. Each time he discarded a worn coat, he stitched a secret pocket into his new coat to conceal this parchment.[21]

Although not immediately, soon enough, Pascal joined an austere religious order, the Jansenists. This group was unworldy in the extreme, and told its members to drop any worldly interests. When Pascal's younger sister became a novice, she already had a career as a poet. The order told her to drop such indulgences. The mother superior, Mère Agnès, "persuaded her not to continue but rather to hide her talent. 'You should hate your genius,' she wrote to her. Jacqueline gave up poetry."[22] When Pascal joined the order, he was likewise told to drop such frivolities as founding new science. He was told to throw out his books, excepting the Bible. He did so.

Some readers might be aghast that a scientific career that might have given birth to even more significant discoveries was nipped. Others might wonder at the ways of spirituality. However, few might expect the aftermath. Pascal composed what are arguably the two greatest religious books of the century. What is unarguable is that they stand *among* (and some critics rate them as *above*) the greatest masterpieces of French prose ever composed.

All this may seem as far from our topic as could be, but think of the question of paradigm shift. In the seventeenth century, building on the work of the Renaissance, there was a massive change in world view underway. For science, it meant a shift from a field that was controlled by religion (with the Bible consulted at every turn) to one that was guided by experiment and reality-testing.

We can see that Pascal proceeded, as it were, backward through this change, first being in the forefront of advancing the experimental perspective, then jumping back to defend the religious view he had been subverting. However, what makes him crucial is not his trajectory but his position in the unstable time of paradigm shift upon which he was to make invaluable observations. Since we, too, are in the midst of such a shift within medicine, trailing a change that has already taken place in physics and certain other sciences, we can benefit from his thoughts, paradoxical as his life may seem to be.

THE CORE OF THIS BOOK

The current bioterrorist threat along with the appearance of hardier forms of older diseases calls for a reliable reference advising in a clear, concise way of simple natural measures that can be taken to enhance your safety, protect your loved ones, and guard your community. The book begins by presenting the pathogens and the diseases they cause, then traditional preventive and therapeutic methods, such as vaccinations and antibiotics, are discussed with their benefits and side effects. Particular attention is paid to the short-falls of vaccines, which have been oversold. This is to say, vaccines' health hazards, both in terms of widespread adverse reactions and (in the case of childhood vaccinations) the overall detriment to immunity involved in the one-sided development encouraged by inoculations, have been little discussed; while vaccines' reputed triumphs in conquering infectious disease have been exaggerated.

Next, natural alternatives to the traditional route are offered, including nutritional supplements. Benefits and side effects of these alternative methods are discussed to enable you to make an informed decision about what is best for your health. First, detoxification guidelines are offered to boost your natural immunity, and to prepare you to receive the greatest absorptive benefit from your therapy of choice. Then the importance of blood pH in maintaining health is presented, together with simple tips on how to create a more alkaline inner environment where microorganisms will replicate with more difficulty. The role of stress reduction in preventing diseases is emphasized, together with simple stress-reducing techniques. A detailed description of herbs and nutrients with immune-enhancing and anti-microbial activity will be presented, to offer you an alternative therapeutic arsenal to be used alone or in conjunction with conventional treatments, in the prevention and treatment of diseases caused by biological agents. Finally, some alternative therapies that tie in with themes to be developed of the collective and democratic bases of health will be highlighted.

We end with further reflections on the public health and community empowerment, explaining how improving your own health is intimately related to compassion for others and taking action to make the community of which you are a part move toward greater well-being.

PART I

BIOLOGICAL WARFARE AND

DRUG-RESISTANT GERMS

History and Perspectives

B iological warfare (BW) is the deliberate use of microbes or toxins to in-
jure or destroy people, animals, or crops through direct measures, such
as aerosol spraying, or indirectly through pollution of water or other resources. Drug-resistant germs are those new strains being promoted by misuse of antibiotics, which often arise in improperly sanitized hospitals. Born
in different parts of the planet, these germs, following the contours of global
travel routes, can make quick transit across seas and continents, thus posing
threats to every nation, regardless of their place of origin.

By way of background, it might be useful to refer back to some key incidents in the appearance of drug-resistant germs and of the use of biological
warfare methods. BW, of course, has a much hoarier history. After all, drug-
resistant germs couldn't appear until there were drugs. In other words, in the
nineteenth century Koch, Pasteur, and their peers discovered that diseases
were caused by bacteria and viruses rather than by bad air, witchcraft or any
of medicine's previous explanations. Only based on this understanding
could drugs and vaccines be produced that would harry germs to such an
extent that the bugs would have to evolve in a particular direction to escape
destruction.

Since histories of biowarfare and, to a lesser extent, of drug-resistant
pathogens, are readily available, appearing especially as the first chapters in
various books on BW, we will eschew elaborate coverage and concentrate on

a few incidents, which will be used to point up the complexity of the field. Of especial note in looking at BW is seeing how difficult it is to decide whether a disease outbreak is planned by an enemy or simply a natural occurrence.

FOURTEENTH CENTURY

One of the most commonly cited early incidents of BW use, although simpler forms of poisoning are traced all the way back to 400 BCE, came in the fourteenth-century siege of Kaffa (Ukraine) by the nomadic Tartars. It is reported the besiegers flung the cadavers of their soldiers who had died from the plague over the walls of the barricaded city. An outbreak of plague followed, with destruction of the city's army. However, an overview in a *JAMA* (*Journal of the American Medical Association*) publication points out that this report is unduly credulous. "Since plague-transmitting fleas leave cadavers to parasitize living hosts, we would suggest that the corpses catapulted over the walls of Kaffa may not have been carrying competent plague vectors."[1] It's more likely that plague arose independently in the city, though the Tartars busily congratulated themselves on the causing it.

NINETEENTH CENTURY

As noted, once the titans of nineteenth-century medicine connected germs to disease and began identifying the particular culpable bacteria and viruses behind different diseases, it became possible to utilize these findings for good or ill. Doctors like the German Koch would develop ways to cultivate these germs in the laboratory as a way to identify illnesses. In his postulates for identifying viruses, Koch laid down that to truly know that a particular virus was present, one would have to isolate it from a patient's blood and then get it to proliferate in a laboratory medium. But once a technique for isolating viruses and bacteria was perfected, these medical gains could be perverted by the military who saw the ability to grow disease agents not as a way to cope with sickness, but as a first step in mass-producing and weaponizing pathogens so as to use them for deviltry on the battlefield.

WORLD WAR I

It was no coincidence, then, that in World War I, Germans led in developing anthrax, cholera, glanders, and a wheat fungus to infect livestock and contaminate animal feed to be exported to Allied forces. They were the farthest ahead in the positive medical advances in isolating disease microbes and viruses, and so could move to the cutting edge in developing military uses of these agents. One saw the same situation in the next world war, when imported German scientists did most of the intellectual work in developing atomic weapons, since it was in their country, led by Einstein and others, that the greatest progress had been made in physics.

However, during World War I, it was *chemical* killing agents, such as the legendary mustard gas, which caused the most shock, devastation and backlash. After the war, the revulsion against these chemical weapons, which had been used by both sides, was such that all the nations involved in the war signed the Geneva Protocol in 1925. This treaty rather myopically forbid the use of chemical and bioweapons but not research, production, and possession of them.

WORLD WAR II

Although biological weapons were not used in the Western theater of war, it appears they were made use of by the Japanese in their conquest of China. "Plague was allegedly developed as a biological weapon by allowing laboratory-bred fleas to feed on plague-infected rats."[2] These fleas were then dropped from planes onto Chinese cities. Each bombardment contained 15 million fleas. The Japanese experience, though, also testifies to the drawbacks of biological weapons. The dispersal of these weapons depends on weather conditions and can backfire by infecting the user's own troops through a shift in the winds or other mishaps. In a 1941 attack by the Japanese on the Chinese city of Changteh where biological weapons were deployed by the invaders, the pathogens ended up killing 1,700 of Japan's own troops and immobilizing another 10,000.

POSTWAR

However, these Japanese attacks as well as the nation's inhuman medical experiments in their prisoner of war camps were not publicly revealed until decades later, and, even then, they received far less publicity than Nazi concentration camp activity.

In consequence, the same type of reaction against chemical and biological weaponry as occurred after the First World War did not appear after the second. Postbellum, all the nations that could afford to went on happily experimenting with biological weapons.

Our own efforts were centered at Camp Detrick, Maryland, and testing sites in Mississippi and Utah. The most worrisome incident in our use of these weapons occurred in trial runs that were carried out through the 1950s and most of the 1960s to assess our nation's vulnerability to germ attack. New York City, San Francisco, and other American cities were covertly exposed to simulants of the aerosolized germs *Aspergillus fumigatus, B subtilis var globigii,* and *Serratia marcescens.* Most devastatingly, an outbreak of infections caused by *S marcescens* occurred at Stanford University Hospital after covert experiments performed in the San Francisco area. Eleven people got sick from the usually benign bacteria, and one of them died. However, although the timing of the people falling sick right after the pathogens were released is suspicious, it has never been possible to prove a direct connection between the experiments and the infections.

1969

In 1969, under pressure because the Vietnam War was going badly and was eliciting increasing protests from the public, President Nixon terminated the U.S's offensive BW program for microorganisms. While most reports explain Nixon's decision in terms of domestic politics, *JAMA* notes that "while many welcomed the termination of the United States offensive program for moral and ethical reasons, the decision…was motivated by pragmatic considerations."[3] It was felt by the military that the arsenal of conventional, nuclear, and chemical weapons was sufficient for all exigencies, and that bioweapons were both unproven and could potentially boomerang. It might be added that delivery systems were still in their infancy and, given that they couldn't be tested, possibly unworkable. It should also be borne in mind that what was closed down by Nixon was *offensive* capabilities. The United States continued with a scaled-back program to look into defense against attack. As critics would charge, this sometimes meant developing the same weapons an offensive program would have created since the defenders felt they had to first create the improved germs their enemies were probably growing before they made protections against them.

JULY 1976

Members of the American Legion sharing a hotel in Philadelphia where they had come for the Bicentennial celebration were infected with a previously unknown bacteria, *Legionella,* which spreads through the air conditioning. One hundred and eighty-two became sick and twenty-nine died. Eventually, scientists found that this pathogen "was a scum bacterium that grew in the biofilms that formed at the interfaces of air and nonsalty water."[4] Such things as infrequently cleaned air conditioners, showers, and dehumidifiers were ideal harbors for this germ.

MID-1970S

A new, extremely deadly form of *Staphylococcus aureus* bacteria appeared in the mid-1970s, striking nearly 400 women (and a few men), killing forty. The disease resulting from the infection was called toxic shock syndrome and surfaced when the invading bacteria so upset the immune system that the victim died of shock. Most of those stricken were women, since the pathogen was fostered by a new type of extended-wear tampon. The bacteria grew inside these feminine products, then issued out to poison the wearer.

SEPTEMBER 1981

At a speech in Berlin, Secretary of State Alexander Haig accused the governments of Kampuchea, Laos, and Afghanistan of using chemical weapons supplied by Russia to kill dissident tribesmen.[5] It was said that three mycotoxins were combined in a yellow rain that was sprayed on rebel encampments. A mycotoxin, a poison derived from a fungus, actually sits on the borderline between chemical and biological weapons. Like a chemical weapon, this substance does not cause a disease but kills or sickens due to its toxin nature. Like a biological weapon, it is a natural product and not the creation of a laboratory.

Also like a biological weapon, it is difficult to determine whether its appearance is planned or natural. In this case, the samples of the yellow rain analyzed consisted largely of pollen. When confronted with the fact that this material didn't seem to consist of scientific preparations of death-dealing poison, but plant extrusions, "the United States Department of State officials...suggested the Russians are using pollen deliberately as a vehicle for transmitting the mycotoxins."[6] The officials also said that pollen would never naturally have fungal toxins piggybacking on it. This point was countered by critics who cited an old study by German and American pathologists, which showed that disease-producing fungi could be carried on pollen grains from infected banana plants to healthy ones."[7]

All of this indicates the peculiarly treacherous nature of biological weapons. Unlike chemical, nuclear or conventional arms, it is hard to know if they have been used and disease casualties have been provoked deliberately. For instance, in trying to track down the truth about yellow rain by interviewing Hmong refugees from the battlefields in Laos—no journalists were allowed close to the war zone—one doctor believes that

> because of the relative lack of sophistication of the Hmong people, any deaths from malaria or haemorragic fevers—both of which occur as local health problems—may be attributed to the chance passing of a MIG aircraft [which it was thought had sprayed the rain, although the actual spraying was not witnessed.[8]

SEPTEMBER AND OCTOBER 1984

The first case of biological terrorism that occurred in the United States came in fall 1984 when 751 people were infected with *Salmonella typhimurium* after an extremist group among the followers of Bhagwan Shree Rajneesh contaminated restaurant salad bars in Oregon.

The Indian spiritual leader Rajneesh attracted many devoted, educated American followers. Having to leave Poona, India, under a cloud of allegations of drug dealing and other illegal actions, in 1981 his group bought a ranch in Wasco County, Oregon. They turned this land into a town called Rajneeshpuram, which in three years had dozen of homes, a shopping mall, a disco, and a 160-room hotel. This town developed its own police force and government. Not satisfied with this extension of their rule, the followers colonized the nearby small town of Antelope, sending in enough new residents to dominate the town council.

Their next plan was to take over the county. The group set up a Share-A-Home program, whereby they brought in 3,000 homeless people from New York and other large cities. Ostensibly a humanitarian effort, the real reason for Rajneeshpuram's largesse was to import pliable voters in hopes of dominating the November 1984 elections. At the same time, under the direction of Diane Onang (Ma Anand Puja), an American nurse born in the Philippines, who was the health officer for the commune, and who had grabbed de facto leadership of the city, where Rajneesh himself did not reside, it was decided that right before the elections a large part of the non-Rajneeshpuram populace in the county would be food poisoned so they would be immobilized and unable to vote. The group's September-October contamination of salad bars was a trial run for a more massive effort scheduled immediately before the election.

As it was, their plans were foiled. When the election approached,

> county officials, citing the large number of registration
> cards [for the upcoming election], insisted that all prospec-
> tive new voters be questioned by a special panel. Realizing
> the homeless would never be able to pass such scrutiny, the
> cult abandoned both the poisonings and the registration
> schemes.[9]

Significantly, the health department attributed the multiple cases of food poisonings to unhygenic conditions at the salad bars, and it wasn't until a year later that the terrorist nature of the episode was discovered and that through accusations of monkey business coming from Rajneesh himself rather than from independent investigation.

This again points up the difficulty of knowing whether a biological attack has really occurred.

SEPTEMBER 1994

In September 1994 cases of plague began to appear in Surat, India, and two-thirds of the population, 500,000 people, fled the city in a week.

Plague had last appeared in India almost thirty years before, and most assumed it had been permanently eliminated. The trouble was this. The *Yersinia pestis* bacteria, which causes the disease, can survive in soil for extended periods. In 1993, Surat was devastated by an earthquake. "Some ten thousand villages were obliterated, one million homes destroyed, and more than ten thousand people killed."[10] It is possible the turnover of the land uncovered buried bacteria. As it was, people quickly moved back into the city, which now lacked adequate housing, water, and other essential services, and had had its medical services severely disarranged.

Although the disease was contained, the panic that had emptied the town testified to a dangerous state of affairs. Some of the people fleeing might have been plague-flea carriers, and if they had been, the sickness would have quickly spread across the whole subcontinent and even the world through long-distance flights. Much of the world reacted by closing its border to Indians and even Indian products. Overall, the Indian and global reactions testify to improvisation, chaos, and lack of foresight, which hardly bode well for coping with the next epidemic.

1995

People in Kikwit, Zaire, began coming down with Ebola fever. This disease is one of the most fearsome known to man, both because of the gruesome way the sufferers die, spewing blood from eyes, mouth, ears, anus, and even through the skin, and because its manner of transmission has not been uncovered.

WHO doctors came forward to help local physicians control the threat. Most chillingly, it was discovered that the disease was spread by unhygienic practices at the hospital. These practices were not a case of sloppiness on the part of personnel, but because the facility was starved for supplies: lacking gloves, sterilizing equipment, and even electricity.[11]

SEPTEMBER–OCTOBER 2001

To bring this brief overview to a close, we might recall a dark page from more recent times. On September 18, 2001, an assistant to NBC news anchorman Tom Brokaw handed a letter to him that turned out to be filled with anthrax spores. A week later the assistant found a raised lesion on her chest, and in the following days began to suffer from headaches, unusual skin redness, and edema. Doctors diagnosed her as suffering from cutaneous anthrax.

She was the first in a series of cases of exposure to the spores, and although she recovered after taking antibiotics, others were not so lucky. Among those dying from the disease were Robert Stevens, who worked at a publishing company which received a tainted letter, and a number of postal employees who presumably handled deadly mail.[12]

> From our survey, it should be evident that there is no dearth of chilling disease challenges, either naturally occurring or concocted by terrorist organizations, peering over the horizon as we move into a new century.[13]

Everything is in place to insure that the assaults of these pathogens will not let up. For one thing, our historical review of the use of biological weapons suggests that interest in implementing and developing bioweapons is likely to continue into the future.

As Osterholm notes, biological agents are the weapons of choice for terrorists. When selecting a weapon, four criteria are worth considering, he writes. In each category, bioweapons win hands down.

First to consider is price. While nuclear weapon production demands a "large, expensive, physical plant," and even chemical weapons have to be created in "an elaborate refinery," biological weapon production "can be set in a typical suburban basement, using basic high school or college lab equipment and materials easily ordered from catalogs."[14]

Bioweapons are also noteworthy for the size of the "footprint" (numbers killed) they can leave. Using an often-cited prediction, it has been noted that twenty-two pounds of anthrax spores dispersed over a large city from a light airplane on a windless day would kill one to three million people. Compare this to a hydrogen bomb, which would murder from a half million to 1.9 million.

Thirdly, the release of a contagious disease agent would be "a gift that keeps on giving" in that the originally infected people, say visitors to a shopping mall, would probably have dispersed to different areas where they would make contact with many people before they knew they were infected, thus spreading the illness far beyond the target area.

Lastly, "the delay between the infection and the onset of the disease...will compound the panic and terror" since many who may have been exposed but are not yet sick will not know "if they are already doomed to become part of the mounting death toll."[15]

In addition, recent advances in modern microbiology and delivery-system technologies have given to bioweapons the potential to impact regional and global security. Progress will likely create an ever-increasing number of deadly mutant microorganisms, which we have the science to produce, without the wisdom nor the technology to control. Currently seventeen countries are suspected of having an offensive BW program.

Further, for all the interlacing reasons connected to failing or neglected public health infrastructures, poor sanitation, abuse of antibiotics, decline in childhood healthcare, the easy movement of illnesses across the world, and other factors we have mentioned, there is bound to be an increase in new drug-resistant viruses and bacteria as well as the resurgence of once moribund illnesses.

Let us look at what diseases are likely to be involved in the coming dismal period.

Biological Weapons

It so happens that most of the disease we have already mentioned as posing dangers because they are developing unmanageable strains or coming back from the dead, diseases such as plague, smallpox, *Staphylococcus,* and Ebola virus, are also on the list of potential biological terrorism agents composed by the Centers for Disease Control and Prevention (CDC), so we can use this list for both prongs of our topic. We will arrange this section according to the CDC's classification.

This grouping of diseases was composed at a meeting held on June 3–4, 1999, at which experts on infectious diseases, public health workers, Department of Health and Human Services (DHHS) officials, and members of the law enforcement, military, and intelligence communities got together to decide on priorities. A three-part division was decided upon, by which biological agents were categorized depending upon (1) their potential impact if released; (2) the ease with which they could be converted into weapons, released on a population and then further spread person to person; (3) "public perception as related to public fear and potential civil disruption," and (4) the public health system's present capabilities to respond to a germ agent release.[16]

The most dangerous agent list, category A, consists of six killers that have "the greatest potential for adverse public health impact with mass casualties" and which would "require broad-based public health preparedness efforts."[17] On this list are anthrax, botulism, plague, smallpox, tularemia, and viral hemorrhagic fevers (such as Ebola virus). The B category contains six pathogens that would also have a devastating impact but would result in less casualties and demand less preparedness from the public health services. Here are found brucellosis, epsilon toxin of *Clostridium perfringens*, glanders, Q fever, ricin toxin, and *Staphylococcus entertotoxin* B. In the last division are placed those agents, namely, hantaviruses, drug-resistant tuberculosis, Nipah virus, tickborne encephalitis, tickborne viral hemorrhagic fevers, and yellow fever, which "currently are not believed to pose a high bioterrorism risk to the public but which could emerge as future threats (as scientific understanding of these agents improves)."[18]

Let's begin by looking at how these different germs attack the human system, noting recent episodes where appropriate, and also attending to how human activity has often sponsored their spread.

CATEGORY A

ANTHRAX (*Bacillus anthracis*)

Anthrax is a disease caused by *Bacillus anthracis*, a gram-positive, spore-bearing bacillus. (Gram-positive simply means that it can be stained for microscopic analysis in a certain way.)

This bacteria lives in the soil and is capable of remaining alive in pastures for years as a spore. The spore is the stage of the bacterial life cycle that is usually infective. Herbivore animals, such as horses and cows, may be contaminated while grazing. The spore can pass naturally to humans who handle infected animals or eat infected meat.

A recent case of such naturally occurring infection was seen in August 2001, the first in the United States since 1972. A North Dakota farmer was hit by the disease. He had "participated in the disposal of five cows that had died of anthrax.... He placed chains around the heads and hooves of the animals and moved them to a burial site."[19] Although he wore gloves at all times, four days after the burial, he noticed a bump on his jaw, which turned out to be a symptom of cutanaeous anthrax. This illness occurred in the midst of a animal epidemic that hit the West in 2000. Thirty-two farms were quarantined, and in three months, 157 animals died.

We should emphasize that anthrax is not contagious and cannot be transmitted from person to person.

While the stricken farmer received the bacteria through the skin, the disease can also invade gastrointestinally and inhalationally.

The *cutaneous form* of anthrax is acquired via inoculation of minor skin lesions with spores from contact with infected animals.

A sore develops with a coal-black center. (Hence the name anthrax, after the Greek word for coal, which is also the root for the word "anthracite," a form of coal). In more than 90 percent of the cases of anthrax in human beings, the bacilli remain within the skin sore, inducing considerable swelling around the lesion and bouts of shivering and chills, but little other disability. Bacilli may, however, escape from the sore and spread up a lymph channel to the nearest lymph node where they are usually halted. Only rarely does the germ invade the bloodstream, causing rapidly fatal septicemia, internal bleeding and sometimes, anthrax meningitis.

Intestinal anthrax is a rare and fatal form of the disease that comes from eating the flesh of animals that have died of anthrax. The disorder causes inflammation of the stomach and intestines with ulcers much like the sores that appear in cutaneous anthrax.

A biological attack with this germ would most likely be delivered with aerosolized spores and would result in *inhalational anthrax*. After being inhaled and deposited in the lower airways, spores are swallowed by tissue macrophages (antibodies whose job is to eliminate intruders by surrounding them). The macrophages transport them to hilar and mediastinal lymph nodes. The mediastinum is located in the middle of the chest, and its enlargement is a telltale sign of infection. Such an enlargement, by the way, was visible on the X-ray Dr. Bartlett brought to Johns Hopkins and was not noticed by the radiologists he consulted.

"In the lymph nodes, in a process that can take anywhere from days to weeks, the spores...turn into anthrax bacteria, which begin producing deadly toxins which attack body tissues."[20] The disease begins with fever, malaise, and fatigue. Cough and chest discomfort may be present. This situation may progress to the abrupt onset of severe respiratory distress with labored breathing and a blueing of the skin. Meningitis appears in approximately half of cases. Death follows within twenty-four to thirty-six hours of toxin release.

The CDC recommends that those who think they may have been exposed watch for these symptoms: Fever above 100 degrees; flu-like manifestations, including cough, fatigue, muscle aches, nausea, vomiting, and diarrhea; and a sore, particularly on the face, arm or hands.

We might note that the recent cases of inhalational anthrax brought about by mailborne terrorism show typical symptomatology and highlight the way bioweapons are apt to catch health workers napping. *JAMA* reported on two postal workers from the Brentwood postal facility in Washington,

D.C., who were exposed to anthrax spores. One began suffering flu-like symptoms soon after contact with the spores, but went on working, attributing his weakness to food poisoning. He collapsed at church four days later, but by the time an ambulance arrived, he had recovered and dismissed the paramedics. The next day he felt so sick he went to a hospital's emergency room. He was examined and discharged "with a presumptive diagnosis of gastroenteritis and instructions to see his primary care physician the following day."[21] His stomach pains grew worse, his breathing was labored, and he was sweating profusely. Again he collapsed. When he arrived at the hospital, the doctors had already *heard reports in the media* about other postal workers hospitalized with anthrax and so quickly tested for this disease.

The second patient had also been sent home from the hospital on first presenting with weakness and high fever. The doctors concluded he had a virus. On his second visit, media coverage alerted the doctors to look in the correct direction.

As predicted by bioterrorism experts, the first appearance of patients with seldom-seen illnesses will catch caregivers napping.

It's also worth remembering that the continental United States is not the only place where anti-American bioterrorists may strike. The CDC investigates alleged cases of the biological weapons use from around the world. In the same time period as Brokaw and others were targeted with mailed spores, anthrax "isolates were recovered from the outer surfaces of letters or packages sent…to the United States embassy in Peru."[22] One postal worker who handled these mail items came down with a case of inhalational anthrax.

(Note: We will discuss the treatment of anthrax in Part 2, where we will concentrate on prophylactics that are controversial. Where the treatment is cut and dried or where, as is often the case, there is no treatment, we will mention it in this part.)

BOTULISM (*Clostridium botulinum*)

Clostridium botulinum is a spore-forming, anaerobic bacteria whose natural habitat is soil. Anaerobic germs are those that can live without oxygen. This bacteria produces the botulism toxin which produces illness.

Three forms of naturally occurring human botulism exist: foodborne, wound, and intestinal. Fewer than 200 cases of all forms of botulism are reported annually in the United States. All forms of botulism result from absorption of botulinum toxin into the bloodstream from either a mucosal surface (gut, lung) or a wound. Botulinum toxin does not penetrate intact skin. Foodborne cases occur when a person swallows food that is tainted with the toxin itself. In the other types of illness, the bacteria grows in the wound or intestine and then produces the debilitating toxin as a byproduct of its metabolism.

While the adult form of *intestinal botulism* appears in relation to tainted food and does not involve intestinal growth; the rare infant form of intestinal botulism does involve such development. "For unknown reasons the botulism bacteria is able to grow in their [children's] intestines."[23] In these childhood cases, the bacteria does not enter the body through toxin-contaminated food, but comes from small trace elements of the bacteria, which are found naturally and which would normally be summarily eliminated by the immune system. The most frequent carrier of this bacteria to children is raw honey, and parents are advised not to feed honey to children in their first months of life.

Wound botulism appears when bacterial spores infect cuts. It normally only occurs among people who have weakened immune systems, being frequently found among drug addicts, for example.

Foodborne botulism is the only form that is commonly seen. "One of the most common culprits in food-borne…[cases] is home-canned foods, especially vegetables such as asparagus, green beans, and peppers."[24] FDA writer Luba Vangelova notes that 90 percent of food-related cases between 1976 and 1985 in the United States could be attributed to home-canned foods.

The most likely form of terrorist use of this toxin would be to create a new airborne form of the sickness that could be labeled *inhalational botulism.* This mode of transmission, which does not occur naturally, has been demonstrated experimentally on primates. Moreover, as post–Gulf War examination of Iraqi biological weapons facilities showed, the arming of missiles and shells with anthrax spores to be spread inhalationally was the focus of a well-developed bioweapon program. We might add that the Japan-based Aum Shinrikyo sect, whose most notorious act was the release of sarin gas (a chemical poison) in Tokyo subways in 1995, resulting in dozens of deaths, also experimented with botulism toxin. The group attempted to spray the toxin in downtown Tokyo, luckily without causing any damage because of a mistake in production of the poison.

Botulism occurs when the toxin, whether produced by active bacteria or ingested, "binds to nerve endings at the point where the nerves join muscles." Vangelova continues, "This prevents the nerves from signaling the muscles to contract. The result is weakness and paralysis that descends from the cranium down, affecting, among other things, the muscles that control breathing."[25]

The neurologic signs in naturally occurring foodborne botulism may be preceded by abdominal cramps, nausea, vomiting or diarrhea. Patients with botulism typically have difficulty seeing (double or blurred vision), speaking (slurred speech and a dry mouth) and/or swallowing, but the patients are not confused or mentally dulled by the onset. The poison moves down the body, hitting first shoulders, then upper arms, then lower arms, and so on down the trunk.

It may be mentioned that, though the botulin toxin is fear-inspiring to most, scientists have managed to find a way to use it for human benefit on two diseases of the eye. Both illnesses are the result of excessive muscular contractions. Use of a small dose of the toxin ends this overreaction without interfering with normal eye use.[26] Less seriously, under the trade name Botox, botulin has also been used to eliminate wrinkles. "Treatment involves injecting very small amounts of the purified toxin into wrinkles. Within two or three days, the muscles that produce frown lines lose their ability to contract."[27]

Historically, people died from botulism when they could no longer breathe as soon as the poison paralyzed the muscles connected to respiration. Now mechanical "ventilators" (breathing devices) can keep victims alive. An antitoxin devised from horse serum can be prescribed, which will neutralize toxin that has not already linked to nerve endings. In order to recover, the patient, kept alive by the ventilator, will have to grow new nerve endings to replace the ones taken over by the toxin. This will take several months.

PLAGUE (*Yersinia pestis*)

The etiologic agent of plague, *Yersinia pestis*, is a gram-negative bacillus carried by numerous rodents, including squirrels, chipmunks, prairie dogs and rats. Plague is transmitted to human beings by bites from infected fleas (that have previously feasted on the rodents) or by rats, or, in the case of pneumonic plague only, by close contact with an infected person. The last form is the only contagious one, spread from the infected by droplets breathed out of the lungs. To catch the disease, one would have to be within six feet of the sick person.

Of the three forms of the disease, the most common is *bubonic plague*, which is characterized by raised, swollen lymph glands (called buboes), fever, chills, and weakness. It is the result of rat or flea bite. In this illness, the bacteria gather and proliferate in these nodes, which their multiplication ends up destroying.

Septicemic plague, which is also not contagious, appears when the plague bacteria has entered the blood, whether as a development of bubonic plague or directly from a bite. It presents with "fever, chills, prostration, abdominal pain, shock and bleeding into skin."[28]

The rarest form is *pneunomic plague*, which can be transmitted not only from person to person but from animal to person. (Recent United States cases involve contact with sick cats.) This is the form bioterrorists would probably choose, using an aerosolized plague spray; although, as mentioned in our historical survey, during World War II, a Japanese attack relied on the bubonic form, disseminated through the release of infected fleas.

In pneunomic plague, after an incubation period of two to three days, patients come down with pneumonia, featuring acute production of a bloody sputum. This plague type progresses rapidly, leading to labored breathing, stridor (a harsh, high-pitched respiratory sound), and a bluish discoloration of skin and mucous membranes.

Although the idea that terrorists may make use of plague is frightening enough, equally disquieting is the appearance of drug-resistant strains.

In our historical notes, we stressed the chagrin in 1994 when India saw its first cases of plague in thirty years. We noted that much of the responsibility for the outbreak could be laid at the door of the the Surat healthcare sector, which had been hobbled by the disarray following upon a devastating earthquake. Whenever healthcare deteriorates sufficiently—and world medical care has been on a downward spiral since the 1990s—there are likely to be such small outbreaks of plague. The *New England Journal of Medicine* notes, "More [plague] cases were reported from 1990 through 1994 than in the preceding decade."[29] These numbers include about fifteen cases a year in the United States, mainly due to "the spread of plague in rodents" in the Western United States.

Along with this disturbing trend of the increase of cases comes a potentially more vexing situation. In 1997 doctors in Madagascar reported the case of a sixteen-year-old boy with a multidrug-resistant case of bubonic plague. "This strain of *Y. pestis* was resistant to all first-line antibiotics as well as to the principal alternative drugs for treatment and prophylaxis."[30] So far this is an isolated example, but there is the possibility that the plague strain the boy carried exists in rats, a possibility which would hold devastating consequences for world health.

Historically, the preferred treatment for plague infection has been various antibiotics. For effectiveness, these must be given within twenty-four hours of the appearance of symptoms. Pneumonic plague is almost certainly fatal if the drugs are not given promptly. Streptomycin; if administered early during the disease, has reduced overall plague mortality to the 5 percent to 14 percent range. Gentamicin is not FDA approved for the treatment of plague, but has been used successfully. This drug is widely available, inexpensive, and can be given once daily. Tetracycline and doxycycline also have been used in the treatment and prophylaxis of plague; both are FDA approved for these purposes.

SMALLPOX (*Variola major* virus)

Smallpox, one of the most terrible diseases known to humanity, has two particularly troubling features. It is highly contagious person to person and, once it is contracted, there is no antiviral or other drug that can combat it.

The illness is an acute infectious disease caused by the *variola major* virus. The word "variola" is Latin for "speckled" referring to the rash and lesions, which appear on face, arms and legs in the course of the sickness.

Smallpox is said to have emerged in human populations about 10,000 BCE. The earliest evidence of smallpox is believed to be the vesicular skin lesions of the mummy of Ramses V, who died in Egypt in 1157 BCE. The term *small*pox was first used in Europe in the 15th century to distinguish variola from the *great* pox, that is, syphilis.

Two forms of smallpox are recognized. *Variola major* was the only form known until the end of the nineteenth century. This is the severe form, characterized by an extensive rash, high fever and prostration, and with a fatality rate of 30 percent or above. According to WHO, the last case of naturally acquired *variola major* occurred in Bangladesh in 1975. (Later, we will see that some dispute this claim.)

Variola minor is less severe with a fatality rate of 15 percent or less. After the last natural case of *variola minor* in Somalia in 1977, smallpox was declared eradicated by the WHO.

There is no animal reservoir for variola; however monkeys are susceptible of infection.

This is a key point, on which we need to briefly expand. "Animal reservoirs" become holding zones for bacteria or (most commonly) viruses. Normally, the animals are not harmed by the germs and are able to pass them on to other creatures. Such reservoirs are essential for long-term germ survival, since if the bugs only affected animals that they rapidly destroyed, they would soon run out of hosts. A virus, such as variola, which does not have an animal reservoir, can be wiped out by heroic public health efforts. By contrast, viruses that have reservoirs, such as the one that causes yellow fever and is spread by mosquitoes, will demand a much greater and riskier effort since to beat the disease would mean exterminating the carrier species.

Variola virus belongs to the family of Poxviridae. In size, these are the largest animal viruses known, being larger than many bacteria and possessing a double stranded DNA genome. Most viruses have only one strand of DNA or RNA. They can remain viable for several days outside a host. In temperate climates, scabs from patients can retain viable virus for several years when held at room temperature.

Smallpox infection begins when the virus comes into contact with the throat or lung mucosa. Virus multiplication then occurs in regional lymph nodes. Lesions appear in the mouth and throat, "releasing large amounts of the virus into the saliva."[31] This accounts for the high contagiousness of the disease, since the affected person releases saliva droplets into the air, which are breathed in by anyone nearby, carrying the virus into the new victim's throat and lungs. Smallpox does not attack internal organs, but confines its work to the skin, blood and respiratory system. The patient dies from toxemia, that is, poisoning due to an abundance of viral toxins in the blood.

There are four clinical presentations of *variola major*, based on the nature and evolution of the lesions. These are not distinctive forms of the disease but differentiations based on the vigor of immune response against the invader.

The most frequent form is *ordinary smallpox*, amounting to 90 percent of cases. *Modified smallpox* is milder and occurs in previously vaccinated people. *Flat* and *hemorrhagic smallpox* are very severe but uncommon variants.

The incubation period of smallpox is twelve days. During this period the patient is well and not infectious. The pre-eruptive stage of the illness begins abruptly, with fever, malaise, headache, muscle pain, prostration and often nausea, vomiting and backache. Temperature usually rises to at least 101° F, often higher. The person is quite sick. This strongly debilitating onset prior to rash occurrence is characteristic of smallpox, and helps differentiate it from many other causes of rash illness.

By the third or fourth day of illness, the temperature usually falls and the patient may feel better. This is the time when the first visible lesions appear and the person becomes infectious. The lesions appear as minute red spots on the tongue, mouth, and throat that become visible about twenty-four hours before the skin rash. The skin rash begins as a few blurred spots on the face. Then the spots spread to the extremities, at first near their connections to the trunk. Usually the rash involves all parts of the body within twenty-four hours. These rashes eventually evolve into raised pustules, usually round, tense, and firm to the touch. These then scab and fall off, often leaving disfiguring scars.

In *modified smallpox*, the first-stage illness is of less force, usually with no fever during the evolution of the rash. The rare *flat-type smallpox* is so named because the lesions remain more or less flush with the skin at the time when raised vesicles form in ordinary smallpox. The fever remains elevated throughout the course of the illness and the patient has severe toxic symptoms. *Hemorrhagic smallpox* involves extensive bleeding into the skin, mucous membranes, and gastrointestinal tract.

The most common rash illness likely to be confused with smallpox is chickenpox. But unlike patients with smallpox who have fever and other symptoms "prodrome," that is, before the onset of the disease in its characteristic form, persons affected by chickenpox have a short, mild prodrome, or no prodrome at all before onset of the rash. Another important distinction between smallpox and chickenpox is the type of rash; smallpox lesions are deep in the skin, round, well circumscribed and hard to the touch, while the chickenpox rash is superficial and not as well circumscribed.

The aerosol infectivity, high mortality, and stability of variola make it a potential threat in BW and terrorism scenarios. Some have argued, however, that smallpox would have limited potential as a biological weapon. Jonathan Tucker, director of Chemical and Biological Weapons Nonproliferation Program at Monterey Institute of International Studies, asserts, "The number of groups that could use smallpox is very, very small," because the ability to weaponize and then deliver this particular virus calls for a high degree of technical expertise." Moreover, he goes on, "They [terrorists] need a motive to cause widespread destruction."[32]

This last point has two connotations. For one, the use of smallpox would not be appropriate for a group with limited political objectives, who was seeking to chastise one country, for example, because a smallpox epidemic would be likely to decimate not one nation state but the whole world. Dr. Donald Henderson, who ran the WHO program that eradicated smallpox, points out that if there were a new outbreak, "to vaccinate all people with whom the patients had had face-to-face contact would be more difficult than it was thirty years ago in Africa and on the Indian subcontinent, where most people still traveled on foot."[33] With the ease and growing frequency of jetsetting, a smallpox attack, which at first would be unidentified, would probably be scattered everywhere before detected. As Henderson puts it,

"With air travel what it is today," the outbreak of smallpox anywhere would be "a global catastrophe."[34]

The second significant problem for would-be smallpox-spreaders follows from what we have just said. Not only would a release of the variola virus affect more than one country, it would probably end up boomeranging and destroying the terrorist's home country. However, even this may not dissuade some groups, such as the sarin-gas-toting Aum Shinrikyo cult, mentioned earlier. Their apocalyptic viewpoint centered on a belief that god wanted the world to end, and it was their role to help bring this about. Such ideas, carried out to their fullest extent, would not blanch at using a disease that would wreak such havoc.

As we know, the first vaccine ever developed was for smallpox, and controversy has swirled around it ever since. We will discuss the vaccine and other traditional prophylactic measures at length in Part 2.

TULAREMIA *(Francisella tularensis)*

Francisella tularensis, the etiologic agent of tularemia, is, to use medical jargon, a small, aerobic facultative, intracellular bacteria. By "aerobic," we mean the microbe needs oxygen to exist; by "facultative," that this bacteria can exist in a number of quite different environments, and by "intracelluar," that, like all viruses but unlike most bacteria, this germ lives inside the cells of its host.

The disease is also called rabbit fever since it is most associated with spread to humans via this animal. In the United States, the disease is normally found where the rabbit carriers reside, particularly in Oklahoma, Arkansas, and Missouri. Early in the twentieth century, it moved East with its host. An article by Katherine Feldman, et al. In the *New England Journal of Medicine* notes, "Cottontail rabbits from Arkansas and Missouri were introduced to Cape Cod and Martha's Vineyard...by game clubs in the late 1930s, and the first locally acquired cases of tularemia were reported shortly thereafter."[35]

Humans acquire the disease through inoculation of skin or mucous membranes with blood or tissue fluids of infected animals or by bites of infected deer flies, mosquitoes, or ticks. Although less common, inhaling contaminated dust or ingesting contaminated foods or water may also produce clinical disease. "Traditionally, hunters, farmers, trappers and butchers became infected" through these means."[36] The virus can remain viable for weeks in water, soil, carcasses and hides, and for years in frozen rabbit meat.

As with the other diseases mentioned, terrorist or military attacks would probably rely on an aerosolized form of the bacteria. Although this form does not often occur, natural flare-ups have happened quite recently, the largest of them was seen in Sweden between 1966 and 1967. "The outbreak involved more than 600 patients infected with strains of the milder European [bacteria]...most of whom acquired infection while doing farm work...when rodent-infested hay was being sorted and moved," casting up aerosolized organisms.[37] Closer to home, fifteen cases were contracted during the summer of 2000 on Martha's Vineyard. Patients were found to have "used a lawn mower or brush cutter in the two weeks before the illness," suggesting their sicknesses derived from bacteria left in the soil by passing animals and then kicked up by the patients' gardening.[38]

Tularemia is commonly divided into two forms in humans, depending on the route of inoculation: ulceroglandular or typhoidal. The more common *ulceroglandular form* is acquired through contact of the skin or mucous membranes with blood or tissue fluids of infected animals. At the onset of illness, there is an elevation of the skin, which is tender and scabbed, at the site of the inoculation. Lymph nodes swell and the sufferer experiences fever, chills, headache and general malaise.

The *typhoidal form*, which occurs mainly after inhalation of infectious aerosols, accounts for from 5 percent to 15 percent of natural cases. Typhoidal tularemia manifests as fever, prostration and weight loss, but without enlargement of the lymph nodes. Respiratory symptoms such as a cough may also be present. Radiological evidence of pneumonia, with associated fluid in the lungs, may be present in all forms of tularemia, but is most common with typhoidal disease. The fatality rate for untreated typhoidal tularemia is approximately 35 percent.

The method of action of this bacteria is to multiply within macrophages (as does anthrax). Its first target is the lymph nodes, but it will also multiply in the lungs, spleen, liver, and kidneys. If the bacteria is not contained by drugs or the patient's immune system, it will eventuate in necrosis, that is, the killing off of individual organs.

The antibiotic streptomycin is the traditional treatment of choice. Gentamicin also is effective. Tetracycline and chloramphenicol are effective as well, but are associated with significant relapse rates.

In the 1930s, the Russians used a live, but weakened form of the bacteria as a vaccination tool to be used on those in tularemia-infested parts of the Soviet Union. A similar vaccine has been used in the United States to inoculate lab workers who came in contact with the bacteria. This drug "is currently under review by the Food and Drug Administration."[39]

VIRAL HEMORRHAGIC FEVERS (VHF) SYNDROME

"Viral hemorrhagic fever (VHF) syndrome" is an umbrella term referring to a string of diseases that have usually been found in the tropics and are characterized by fever, prostration and problems with circulation, including permeability of the blood vessels whereby blood seeps out into the surrounding tissue. Some of these diseases are *new* to humans, which, as we will see, does not mean that the virus itself is novel, but simply that it never previously crossed from its animal hosts to our species.

Despite their diverse taxonomy, the VHF agents are typically transmitted to humans by contact with infected animals, whose distributions tend to determine the geographic ranges of these diseases. Tickborne hemorrhagic fever viruses, for example, which include a number of different viruses to be mentioned here, stay within the range of their tick hosts, commonly striking in the seasons when those insects are the most active. (Note: we will discuss the tickborne fevers in passing here in order to deal with all the VHFs in the same section, although technically they belong in Category C.)

Many of the VHFs, such as Argentine hemorrhagic fever and Rift Valley fever, get their names from the locale in which they are typically or were first found. As we will explore, recent changes in human demographics that have altered animal habitats have increased human exposures to these viruses. In addition to natural disease potential, many of the VHF agents are potential BW threats as well. These viruses are highly infectious by aerosol; are associated, in some cases, with high mortality; and may replicate sufficiently well in cell culture to permit weaponization.

The VHF causers are all RNA viruses. This means simply that the virus, a rather simple structure that consists of nucleic material and a containing envelope, has RNA rather than DNA inside its skin. We may mention that unlike bacteria, which are living things, viruses do not function apart from host cells. A virus, once on board its prey, will float around the blood until it locks onto a cell. Then the envelope operates to automatically inject its RNA or DNA inside. Within the cell, the viral program, inscribed in the nucleotide strands, commandeers host machinery to help it reproduce. Thus, it can only become active with the help of what it is parasiting.

VHF is associated with viruses from four families: *Arenaviridae*, including viruses that produce Lassa fever, Argentine hemorrhagic fever, and Bolivian hemorrhagic fever; *Bunyaviridae*, associated with Crimean-Congo fever and the Hanta viruses; *Filoviridae*, connected to Ebola and Marburg viruses; and finally *Flaviviridae*, which includes the yellow-fever producing virus.

Patients with VHF generally benefit from rapid, nontraumatic hospitalization to prevent unnecessary damage to the fragile capillary bed. Secondary infections are common and should be sought and treated aggressively. The management of bleeding is subject to controversy. In the absence of definitive evidence, it is recommended that mild bleeding manifestations not be treated at all. Ribavirin is of proven value for some, but not all of the VHF agents.

Now let's look at some of the specific viral illnesses in more detail.

THE ARENAVIRIDAE

LASSA FEVER

This disease was first noticed by Western observers in 1969 and named for a village in Eastern Nigeria where the first official case was seen. The victim was nurse Laura Wine of the Church of the Brethren hospital. When local treatment proved futile, she was flown to the nearest large town, Jos, where she died in the hospital. Then nurses and missionaries who treated her began to come down with this previously unknown illness, which racks the body with fever, chest pains, vomiting, diarrhea, bleeding gums and other disturbances. One stricken Jos nurse, Lily Pinneo, was flown to New York City with tissue and blood samples to see whether American doctors could block the diseases that so far were generally leading to painful deaths in which the victim went into convulsions.

Autopsies indicated those who died from Lassa fever had every organ devastated by the virus, with fluid and blood in the lungs, the heart clogged, and the liver and spleen filled with dead cells. Pinneo managed to beat the disease, though this was due to a hardy immune system rather than anything the doctors could do. However, in the meantime Dr. Jordi Casals at Yale, who was analyzing patients' tissue blood, came down with the disease. He managed to beat it, too; but one of his lab assistants died from the illness. Casals couldn't figure out how he or his worker were infected, and the situation was so alarming to the university that it closed down the research laboratory.[40]

One frightening thing about this disease is that it seems to pass so easily from person to person, although it originally enters a human community by way of its animal reservoir, the multimammate rat (*Mastomys natalensis*). These rats live in the forests and savannas of West, Central, and East Africa, and scurry through village homes looking for food. Once the disease has moved from animal to human, it can then go between humans, whether moving through the air, by inhalation of infected particles from a sick person, or by blood to blood contact, such as when someone is stuck with an infected needle.

A change in the ecological balance, though a minor one, seems to have spurred the appearance of the disease. CDC research doctors who came to Nigeria to try and track down how the virus was spreading noted that there were two species of rats found in the villages, the *Mastomys* and a larger black rats (*Ratus ratus*). "In some villages, the people had driven out or eaten the big black rats, leaving smaller brown Mastomys virtually unopposed on the playing field."[41] Where the multimammate rats' competitor was eliminated, and thus where more of the culprit rodents were present, seemed to be where the fever would strike.

Early on, the only thing that was found to halt the spread of the virus was transfusing a patient with the blood of someone who had recovered from the illness. Shortly, it was discovered that this was only effective for a few months after the recovery. Traditional medicine prescribes Ribavirin, which seems effective if given early in the sickness. Otherwise, supportive care and treatment of accompanying infections are the best palliatives.

ARGENTINE HEMORRHAGIC FEVER (JUNÍN FEVER)

This fever was first noticed in 1953 near the Junín River in Argentina where it struck down corn harvesters. Its method of destruction was to weaken the capillaries of those infected. So much blood was leaked out that a sufferer bled to death.

Doctors from the Rockefeller Foundation and Buenos Aires University, who worked together to uncover the trajectory of the disease as it went from animal host to human, discovered that this was another case where changes in the ecosystem ripened conditions for the virus's emergence. The corn growers of the region had always been bothered by a short weed, which seemed ineradicable and would clog their fields, lessening the crop yield. Then, after World War II, the agricultural workers obtained pesticides, which they used to eliminate these pesty plants. With this vegetation out of the way, though, there was a gaping hole in the ecological ladder, which was filled by a tall grass. However, this intruder proved less noxious to the farmers since it didn't choke off the growth of their plants. Things seemed to be looking up for corn growers. There was one catch. "As it turned out, a fairly rare species of field mouse subsisted on the seeds of these tall grasses. As the grasses proliferated, so did the mice, until the once-rare species became the dominant rodent of the region."[42] This mouse was the carrier of Junín fever.

Meanwhile, there was a second wrinkle. The scientific team noticed that the villages where fever cases occurred were cat-less. Apparently the DDT used (and overused) to kill the small weeds, also eliminated the felines, and with no cats, the unpoliced mice could proliferate all the faster.[43]

In this case and in that of the next VHF we will study, we are seeing that what purported to be a great ameliorator, the Green Revolution—a strategy by which Western techniques of agriculture, such as heavy use of pesticides and massive growing of a single crop for export, were adopted in underdeveloped countries in place of indigenous methods of crop culture such as growing a diversity of fruits, vegetables and grains—mostly led to disaster.

In fact, the Green Revolution, which was pushed as heavily by Western governments in the 1960s as they are now pushing austerity programs as ways for underdeveloped countries to lower their massive debt loads, proved disastrous. What happened was the new techniques drove peasants out of the countryside into the pesthole slums of port cities. The techniques of the Green Revolution, such as use of pesticides, were extremely expensive and were best employed on large estates. Western foreign aid was used by the rich farmers to buy out the peasants or to hire strong men to drive them away. Even where peasant proprietors were funded to join in the Green Revolution projects, the "improvements" could be counterproductive as when a local ecosystem's inter-balance was smashed and, as in the case we are examining, new diseases are unleashed.

Though the presenting symptoms of Argentine hemorrhagic fever, from the fever to diarrhea and muscle aches, are much like those of the other VHFs, it shares the distinction with yellow fever of being one of the two viral hemorrhagic fevers for which a vaccine has been developed by traditional medicine. Ribavirin can be used to reduce infection and is now used routinely as an adjunct to immune plasma.

BOLIVIAN HEMORRHAGIC FEVER

This disease was first spotted in 1962 in the remote town of Orobayaya in Bolivia. The afflicted were brought low with fever, profuse sweating, fatigue, severe pain, and the leaking of blood from microscopic holes in capillaries. Fatalities appeared—this disease has one of the greatest fatality rates of all the HFVs—when the virus either escalated its attack and broke down the nervous system, whereby muscle spasms were followed by a seizure, or if the leaking blood became so massive the body went into shock.

In 1963 a team from the United States' National Institutes of Health (NIH) investigated this outbreak, and, after a year and a half's work (and after two of the three men involved had caught the fever, which they survived), it was determined the agent spreading initial infection was mouse urine, which was deposited in the adobe houses of the victims.

Bolivian hemorrhagic fever, in the same manner as Junín fever, came to light at this historical juncture due to ecological disruptions pioneered by humans. The situation has been carefully teased out in *The Coming Plague* by Laurie Garrett. As she tells the story, for decades the area in which the disease originated had been focused on cattle raising under the direction of wealthy Brazilian landowners, who also controlled the river boats that took the cattle to market. However, after a 1952 nationalist revolution in Bolivia, the Brazilians had their land expropriated and they subsequently fled, leaving the villagers without the resources to raise and market the cows. They turned to raising cattle for themselves and supplementing this with farming. "in their haste to grow corn and other vegetables, they chopped down dense jungle areas...[and] unwittingly disrupted the natural habitat of the *Calomys* field mouse [host of the Bolivian hemorrhagic fever virus] and provided the rodent with a superior new food source: corn."[44]

Here is another example of a disease coming into the human population as soon as a semi-pristine ecology undergoes a radical alteration, engineered by human activity.

As with smallpox, there are no drug treatments once the disease has gained hold. Supervised bed rest is a necessity as well as monitoring of liquids and electrolytes which need to be boosted due to their outflow through the broken vessels. (We will not include treatment sections below for other VHFs unless suggestions go beyond the above.)

BUNYAVIRIDAE

CRIMEAN-CONGO HEMORRHAGIC FEVER (CCHF)

As the name implies, this viral infection is found in a wide territory, spanning areas in the former Soviet Union and crossing Eastern Europe, Asia, and Africa. Indeed the name itself was created when the near-global reach of the virus was recognized. In 1944, the disease was identified in the Crimea and dubbed Crimean hemorrhagic fever. "In 1969 it was recognized that the pathogen causing Crimean hemorrhagic fever was the same as that responsible for an illness identified in 1956 in the Congo, and linkage of the two place names resulted in the current name for the disease."[45]

The area the viruses cover, as Dr. Bob Swanepoel of the National Institute for Virology in Johannesburg states, "coincides pretty well with the distribution of Hyalomma ticks."[46] This tick is the main reservoir for the viral agent, but it is an insect that only rarely bites humans, preferring to dine on sheep and cows. Humans generally contact the virus through handling of livestock, and the disease is usually found in farm settings. "The only town dwellers who are regularly exposed to infection are slaughter men at abattoirs—since they encounter fresh blood and other tissues of livestock...hundreds of times daily."[47] Curiously, even a worker at an ostrich slaughterhouse once came down with the disease, possibly transmitted from ticks on the birds' pelts.

Animal to human transmission of the fever has been well established, but it has been postulated that human to human transfer also occurs. "The increasing number of cases [that] have occurred among the medical and nursing staff caring for patients in hospitals and in laboratory personnel carrying out investigations of these patients," indicate to James Gear and associates that contact with patients' blood can also pass the virus.[48]

As does Argentine hemorrhagic fever, this illness responds favorably to traditional treatment with ribavirin. Although the majority of the studies of the drug's viral-stemming ability look at ribavirin's effect on the virus in cell cultures, there is one investigation of its action in the field. This was done by S. P. Fisher-Hoch and others and reported in *Lancet* in 1995. The Fisher-Hoch group looked at three health workers in Pakistan who were laid low by CCHF virus, with symptoms of anemia and prostration, and who "all had an estimated probability of death of 90 percent or more."[49] They were given 4 grams of Ribavirin for four days and 2.4. grams for the following six days. The patients completely reversed the drastic decline of their vital signs within two days and all returned to normal health.

THE HANTA VIRUSES

(Note: we have placed the discussion of these viruses here because one of their two major forms produces a hemorrhagic fever, and so it would seem most logical to discussion them in relation to the other VHFs. However, strictly speaking, the CDC does not think it likely that these viruses will be militarized, and so has classified them under Category C.)

These viruses were first recognized during the Korean War when 2,500 American soldiers and many Korean fighters came down with a mysterious fever, which led to weakness and kidney failure. Most of the sufferers recovered, but there were 121 deaths. Eventually the cause of this illness was identified as Korean Hantaan virus. It was transmitted by field mice, who range through Korea, Japan, Northeastern China, and southeastern and Central Russia. Dr. Karl Johnson for the United States Army and Dr. Ho Wang Lee of Korea University Medical Schools hypothesized that the virus emerged at this time "when aerial bombing campaigns drove the A. agrarius field mice out of their natural habitats into urban areas, where they got into turf battles with the rats and probably passed the virus on to the larger rodents during biting and clawing fights."[50]

In the 1970s, other viruses from this same family, which caused similar physical failures and were also carried by rodents, were identified in Eastern Europe and Africa.

It wasn't until 1993 that doctors saw a rash of deaths attributable to a Hanta virus occur in the United States, although earlier biologists, testing American harbor rats in the 1980s, found they carried the Korean Hanta virus. The rats were caught and studied in the first place under Johnson's urging, in that he posited "since Korea was rapidly becoming one of America's biggest trading partners...infected Seoul rats might have found their way into cargo holds of Korean ships and then escaped into United States harbor cities.[51]

The 1993 cases occurred on Indian reservations. A number of young, healthy people succumbed to what seemed inexplicable breathing problems. At first, no one thought these were cases of a Hanta virus, since they cause kidney failure, not the filling of the lungs with fluid which eventuated in death in these cases.

A full-scale investigation was called for and it became one for the books. Not only because, as Garrett explains, of the speed with which the identification of the culprit was achieved, the cordial and supportive relations of the different state and federal agents, and the use of new polymerase chain reaction (PCR) technology, which can quickly isolate different viral proteins in a patient's blood sample; but because of the way the investigation established reciprocal connections with the affected community.

Dr. Jim Cheek, an epidemiologist for the New Mexico Department of Health, put it like this, "We decided to have the Navajo people involved in every step of the investigation. I insisted on it." In Garrett's words, "what followed was an investigation unprecedented in its integration of community members into every aspect of the inquiry."[52] It was the community that clued scientists into what direction to take their inquiry when people noted that good rains had yielded a larger-than-usual crop of piñon nuts and, as a consequence, an explosion of the population of the rats that fed on them. Blood samples of these rats showed the presence of a new Hanta family virus, one that devastated the lungs rather than the kidneys.

At this point, then, biologists began to mark a division in the Hanta viruses between hemorrhagic fever with renal syndrome (HFRS) and hantavirus pulmonary syndrome (HPS). Both are spread by mice. The CDC reports,

"These rodents shed the virus in their urine, droppings, and saliva...when fresh rodent droppings or nesting materials are stirred up...[then] tiny droplets containing the virus get into the air," and are breathed in by humans.[53] Once stricken, a victim feels muscle aches, fever, and fatigue. For HPS, the only form of the disease so far seen in our country, the patient often also experiences headaches, vomiting, diarrhea, and cough.

As to how to deal with cases of HPS, the CDC has this to say, "At the present time, there is no specific treatment or 'cure' for hantavirus infection." The best that can be done is take a patient to an intensive care unit. "In intensive care, patients are intubated and given oxygen therapy to help them through the period of respiratory distress."[54]

FILOVIRIDAE

EBOLA VIRUS

The Ebola virus is the most notorious and most feared of the VHFs. Its notoriety is due to a chance conjuncture of circumstances, while its fearsomeness springs from its killing power and unknown origin.

The first recognized outbreaks of the disease occurred in 1976 in the Sudan and Zaire, hitting 284 and 318 cases, respectively for each country, with 150 and 180 deaths. (Retrospective analyses showed that there had been unrecognized occurrences of this disease as early as the 1960s in Ethiopia.) These alerted the world health community to the emergence of a new, pernicious health threat.

The American people, however, did not become particularly alarmed until there was an outbreak among monkeys in a lab in Reston, Virginia. This itself might not have aroused public fears, except that the whole story was put in a book by science writer Richard Preston. The text, *The Hot Zone*, did all it could to fan the flame of public fears by emphasizing how easily Ebola might have been transferred to an animal handler and then have spread through the state. The book was something of a tour de force in that it told a suspenseful story in which nothing much happened. Not one person got the disease. Later, in fact, it would turn out that this strain of the virus was not transmissible to humans. The story was picked up and fictionalized by Hollywood, and since that time Ebola has resided in the public consciousness.

However, although there is often a wide discrepancy between fears the media is fixated upon and those we should be realistically concerned with, in this case there is a solid foundation for trepidation. For one thing, the disease has proved fatal in the majority of cases. While in the most recent epidemic for which statistics are available, one which took place in Uganda from summer 2000 to winter 2001, of 425 patients, 224 died (a 53 percent mortality rate), in other recent occurrences death has ranged higher, hitting 77 percent in Zaire in 1995. In one of the first noticed outbreaks in 1976 in Zaire, 88 percent of those who caught the disease, succumbed.[55]

As the recent dates of some of these incidents suggest—and there was a further occurrence of the disease in December 2001 in the Congo for which details are not yet available—this disease is far from under control. One of the reasons for this is that no one knows where the disease comes from although we can be fairly sure that there is an animal carrier. In fact, as Dr. John King of Louisiana State University Sciences Center (in an article coauthored with Dr. Anurag Markanday), points out, "To date, no reservoir has been identified for any Filovirus."[56] It is hard to guard against a disease when its source is unknown.

Once one person has contracted the disease, contact with the blood and other fluids of this person has acted to spread it further. King notes, in relation to 1976 Zaire cases,

> admission to hospital acted to greatly amplify the frequency of transmission. The lack of proper barrier protection (gloves, fluid-resistant gowns, and proper sanitation) and the use and reuse of contaminated medical equipment, especially needles and syringes, resulted in rapid nosocomial spread of infection.[57]

One might ask how it is the Ebola flare-ups were always stopped quickly, with the numbers getting sick never going much beyond three hundred, given that what is causing the disease has not been determined and that iatrogenic passing of the disease in medical facilities in the poorer countries is likely to continue? Why has Ebola not spread like a modern-day black plague?

In an close reading of what happened in the 1976 Zaire Ebola episode, Garrett notes that folk knowledge played a large role in heading off disaster. She describes what happened when three emissaries from WHO arrived in the locale of the sickness:

> Everywhere the group went they noticed the people had taken remarkably wise measures to stop the epidemic's spread. Roadblocks were staffed around the clock.... The ailing villagers and their families were kept under quarantine, bodies were buried some distance away from the

houses, and there was little movement of people between communities.… The scientists humbly agreed that their expertise had not been necessary to arrest the epidemic.[58]

The people also had the presence of mind not to send anyone to the hospital since they rightly surmised that people were becoming infected with Ebola under nurses' care.

As with other HFVs, Ebola begins with fever, headache, muscles pains, and weakness. Soon after come gastrointestinal pains, vomiting and diarrhea. There is internal bleeding in the gastrointestinal region as well as from the gums. In last stages, as the virus attacks endothelial cells, which line the blood vessels, more blood leaks, causing such manifestations as the vomiting of blood, and blood leaking from nose, eyes, and other areas.

As of yet, there is no therapy of proven effectiveness against this retrovirus. Ribavirin, which has worked against a number of hemorrhagic fevers, has no effect on Ebola. King reports that four Russian lab workers, who *may* have been infected with the disease, were treated with Ebola antibodies produced by giving goats the disease as well as human interferon, and this seemed to prove effective, though no further study of this combination has been done.[59]

MARBURG VIRUS

We have noticed that the hemorrhagic fever viruses are commonly named for the regions in which the first cases of the disease are recorded, and that this place has been found to coincide with the stamping ground of the virus's animal carrier.

The Marburg virus—Marburg is an industrial city in Germany—matches only one of those criteria. Its first known cases were indeed seen in this European city in 1967, but this is hardly the natural habitat of the vervet monkey, the viral host.

What happened was this. Marburg is the site of a production facility of Behringwerke AG, a German vaccine maker. The first three men hit by the VHF were employees in the plant, who worked with monkeys or monkey tissue. Eventually thirty-one people caught the disease (nine died); and all either worked at this plant, had handled the monkeys in transit from Uganda, or were health workers in contact with the blood of the first patients. Blood workups on the animals brought to light this previously unknown virus.[60]

This is definitely a new wrinkle. Cases such as that of the surfacing of an ultra-resistant strain of TB in New York City that had previously been seen in

Russia was taken to indicate the speed and facility with which germs were moving globally, carried by air passengers. Now, we have to append the further point that not only people but goods, including animals, are circulating in greater numbers and with greater velocity between nations, and this ups the odds of viral and bacterial border-hopping.

However, the discovery of Marburg virus in the monkeys did not solve the problem of where the virus originated in that the monkeys with the virus were dying from it. An animal reservoir, as we have defined it, contains a virus that has no detrimental effects on its host. The reservoir is threatening to others species because it remains robust, carrying the virus until it has time to jump into another type of host.

The Marburg virus, which appears in a virulent and mild form, begins with fever and muscle ache, and then progresses to a swollen spleen and lymph nodes. So far this is not unlike the course of other hemorrhagic fevers. Next, though, the patients are bothered by red rashes, followed by a reddening of the skin due to the blockage of capillaries. With limited blood movement, oxygen is not reaching the cells and they begin to die. The skin begins peeling off the body, while blood loses the ability to coagulate. Eventually a victim suffers brain damage or heart attack.

There are no known effective drugs for treating Marburg, and the best that can be done is isolate the patient and offer supportive care.

FLAVIVIRIDAE

DENGUE FEVER

This last of the hemorrhagic fevers is spread in part by the same mosquito as is urban yellow fever. Thus, its fortunes have been seen to rise and fall along with that other disease, lessening in impact when yellow fever eradication efforts were underway, and springing up again when those efforts have slackened off. This disease has been recorded since the eighteenth century, but, though bothersome since its major symptoms were headaches, eye pains, and joint aches, it was uncomfortable but not disabling or fatal.

However, an outbreak in the Philippines in the early 1950s brought into focus a new strain of the disease, dengue-2, which had a more ferocious impact on the body and a more insidious way of attacking the immune system. Moreover, it was soon found that both dengue types could be spread by more than one type of mosquito.

Dengue-2 fever not only causes aches and pains, but a rash of red spots on the skin (indicative of capillary leakage), high fevers (ones recorded reaching 107° F), shock, and convulsions. This virus's method of attack turns the immune system against itself by commandeering macrophages. These immune system cells surround and stifle intruding microbes. The dengue-2 virus hijacks them, for once it is internalized by the macrophage, it uses the macrophage to carry it to vulnerable parts of the body, sustaining itself inside the immune system cell, which would kill most interlopers. Moreover, it was found that exposure to the milder dengue, primed a person to get a killing dose of dengue-2, since the first case would leave a memory in the body's immune system, making it quicker to call up antibodies. In this case, the more quickly the body responded, sending out macrophages, the more quickly the virus would spread.[61]

The story of the genesis of dengue-2 is yet another powerful illustration of how human backing has been instrumental in developing new disease strains. Before World War II, there were various versions of a mild dengue existing in different parts of the world, with each type staying in a particular eco-locale. Obviously, the war disrupted insect control activities that had been so useful in keeping their numbers low since the days of Walter Reed. Moreover, the mass movements of people, whether troops or refugees, as well as the displacement that left many confined in close quarters in camps, were ideal for the spread of disease. The collapse of mosquito eradication meant a boon for the A. aegypti variety, "which may very well have numbered more in 1945 than at any time in the planet's previous history."[62]

Sick people would move from one theater of war to the other. Infected by one dengue type in one region, a soldier or displaced person might be bitten by a mosquito with another type in a new location. This was not only bad for the sufferer, but for the new area's population because the mosquito would be mixing two dengue types in her gut. (Only the female bites in this species.) Tom Monath of the United States Army's Medical Research Institute of Infectious Disease, argued that dengue-2 first emerged in the Philippines in 1953 because of these wartime dislocations had promoted the cross-pollination of dengue types.

> After a few years of circulation among humans and mosquitoes in Manila, the immune system cycle necessary for the creation...of dengue-2 was in place. Such serial infection of one dengue type after another hadn't been possible been World War II, Monath concluded, because few—if any—areas of Asia had endemic dengue of more than one type.[63]

Another discerning student of how humans have unintentionally inter-acted with viruses in a way that gave them a more menacing profile or spread them more widely is Dr. Duane Gubler of the CDC. He notes that the more virulent form of dengue is spread more easily by the hardier *A. albopi-cutus* (or tiger) mosquito. Luckily, that mosquito species was not native to the United States and so was not a threat...until 1985. "Carried aboard a shipment of water-logged used tires sent from Japan for retreading in Hous-ton," the mosquitoes made their appearance in America. "Within two years...tiger mosquitoes would be seeking human blood in the cities and towns of seventeen U.S. states."[64]

Although dengue fever has not yet appeared on the U.S. mainland, it has cropped up in South America and the Caribbean, carried somehow from its original confinement in the Far East. As with most of the other viral hemor-rhagic fevers, there is no vaccine or antiviral that has shown itself effective against it. The only treatment is bed rest and supportive nursing.

CATEGORY B

The next set of disease we wish to concentrate on are less destructive to the health and less easily weaponized. An examination of them can teach us still more about biological warfare and about the adaptive power of germs.

BRUCELLOSIS

Brucellosis is produced by a small, slow-growing bacteria. Because of its lag-gardly reproductive rate, the time between infection and onset of illness tends to be long and variable, reaching from a week to sixty days. There are six known species of Brucella bacteria, which are closely related, though each characteristically infects a different animal host, whether it be a goat, pig, cow, or dog. It is contact with these hosts that brings disease to an individual.

Brucellosis is also known as Malta fever in remembrance of the fact that it was first identified in the 1850s during the Crimean War when it struck down British soldiers stationed in Malta. It was determined that the men were falling prey to the illness due to consumption of raw goat's milk and cheese. Once they stopped eating and drinking these infected supplies, the incidences of brucelloisis dropped off.

Nowadays, the infection is still brought about mainly through animal contacts. The CDC reports that brucelloisis is "commonly transmitted through abrasions of the skin from handling infected animals. In the United States, [it] occurs most frequently by ingesting contaminated milk or dairy products."[65] It can also be spread through accidental exposure in laboratories when working with animal tissues or blood. Most rarely, it is transmitted by inhalation.

It is this last-mentioned manner of infection that most exercised the United States military, which weaponized the *B. suis* strain of the bacteria in the 1940s and 1950s. It turns out that brucelloisis, though far from one of the nastier diseases that could have been chosen, was one of those on which America's biological warfare unit, newly created during World War II, cut its teeth In its early research with this germ, it learned the importance of miniaturization. By the mid-1950s, "researchers...discovered that the dosage of some forms of brucelloisis required to infect a guinea pig is six hundred times greater with particles of 12-micron size than it is with 1-micron particles." As Seymour Hersh explains, "The very small particles are capable of avoiding the natural body defenses found in the cilia of the nose and upper respiratory tract."[66]

To stay with early United States biological warfare experiments for a moment, we might mention further that brucellosis was a prototype for the mass production of disease which is at the foundation of such programs. To refer to Hersh again, "Researchers at Detrick developed a continuous culture machine capable of producing brucelloisis (Brucella) germs by the ton." This was translated into a paste that held about 25 *trillion* bacteria per ounce. "One ounce was enough to infect more than two billion persons."[67]

As with dengue-2 fever, this germ becomes a parasite on macrophages and eventually localizes in organs (especially the lung, spleen, liver, central nervous system, and bone marrow). Disease manifestations reflect this distribution.

Stricken patients usually suffer from fever, chills, headache, weakness, muscle and joint aches, and malaise. Depression and other psychological changes can also be noted. Endocarditis (inflammation of the heart) and central nervous system infections are rare, but account for nearly all fatalities, which amount to less than 5 percent of untreated patients.

Systemic symptoms may last for weeks or months. Even without treatment, most patients recover within a year, but relapses are common.

A combination of the antibiotics doxycycline and rifampin orally for six weeks is the traditional treatment of choice. Alternative treatments would use cotrimoxazole and gentamicin or ofloxacin and rifampin.

TOXINS OF CLOSTRIDIUM PERFRINGENS

We've seen that, aside from the damage bacterial infection causes when the proliferating germs harm organs and other body parts by overrunning them and gobbling up food and oxygen, the invasive microbes may also harm the host by extruding a toxin, as occurs with anthrax. When one is hit by one of these bacteria, it is as if one had a machine for producing poisons hooked up in one's cells.

The *Clostridium perfringens* bacteria is a germ that produces a debilitating toxin, which is responsible for the most cases of food poisoning in the United States. The FDA's Center for Food Safety and Applied Nutrition's *Bad Bug Book* notes that in 1981, for example,

> [t]here were 1,162 cases [of *Clostridium perfringens* bacteria poisoning]…in twenty-eight separate outbreaks. At least ten to twenty outbreaks have been reported annually in the United States for the past two decades. Typically, dozens or even hundreds of persons are affected.[68]

The reason such large numbers are affected per outbreak is that the food poisonings generally take place in institutions. "In most cases, the actual cause of poisoning by *C. perfringens* is temperature abuse of prepared foods."[69] The food may not have been fully cooked, and so a small amount of bacteria survives. Then, while the food is set aside before being given out in a hospital, school, prison, or other large facility, the bacteria remultiplies.

The *Bad Bug Book* gives as an example of a representative flare-up a case that struck a Connecticut factory in 1985. There 599 employees out of 1,362 came down with the illness, which was later attributed to gravy. "The gravy had been prepared twelve to twenty-four hours before serving, had been improperly cooled, and was reheated shortly before serving."[70]

Sadly enough, one eruption of sickness does not necessarily lead to reform of food-handling practices as another example confirms. In March 1984, seventy-seven prison inmates were infected with the *C. perfringens* bacteria, which was present in roast beef. A week later prisoners at the same jail were caught again by the disease, this time conveyed to them in ham.

We have talked of how current human practices facilitate the spread and improvement of germs, as when disruption of wilderness areas changes the habits of a pathogen reservoir. Another way humans have impacted germ spread is by the increasing use of mass kitchens. In the United States, in particular, more and more people eat in institutions, whether these be boot camps, corporate cafeterias, elementary school lunchrooms or, most significantly, fast food restaurants. With this change, chances of food poisoning skyrocket.

Obviously, one can be fed bacteria in a home-cooked meal. See the skit in Monty Python's *The Meaning of Life*, where a dinner party is wiped out by salmon mousse. However, for a number of reasons, food from fast-food emporiums and other large-bore cookeries are more likely to account for sickness attributable to bad food than are home servings. For one, the heating, cooling down and reheating of comestibles, which are common in institutional kitchens and which foster bacterial growth, are less typically done in the home. Moreover, there is the question of concern. It stands to reason a person making a holiday meal for relatives is going to prepare the courses more carefully than, for example, an underpaid, harried chef at a McDonalds or Wendy's. It's human nature to put more loving attention into a task done for family or intimates than for strangers. Lastly, there is the sheer numerical difference. A family Christmas may involve a score of eaters, while a factory cafeteria, such as the Connecticut one we mentioned, serves more than a thousand at each sitdown. Even if cooks in mass kitchens were as scrupulous as those whipping up a snack for friends, the repercussions of a slip-up in their work will be much greater, leading to a larger per capita sickness.

It wouldn't have taken a sociology degree or a crystal ball to predict that, over the last few decades, as Americans have come to rely more heavily on meals prepared at institutions, more cases of food poisoning would appear. Eric Schlosser, in his recent best-seller *Fast Food Nation*, includes this surprising statistic: "Every day in the United States, roughly 200,000 people are sickened by a food-borne disease, 900 are hospitalized, and fourteen die."[71] He concludes further, "There is strong evidence not only that the incidence of food-related illness has risen in the past few decades, but also that the lasting health consequences of such illnesses are far more serious than was previously believed."[72]

He bases the later claim on evidence from medical studies that show pathogens passed through food can lead, in the long run, to kidney problems, autoimmune dysfunction, heart disease, inflammatory bowel disease, and neurological difficulties. Schlosser ties the origins of this spate of food-borne illness, not to institutional cooking but to an earlier place on the agribusiness pipeline. He feels most germs get into the American diet through the way cattle and other animals are raised and slaughtered.

Still, the principle remains the same. A change in American habits, fueled both by longer working hours and increasingly fragmented families, has shifted eating out of the home. People resort to the mass meal makers, who, because of their own shortcomings or due to the faults of their food suppliers, often serve up pathogens with their dinners. As we've seen, *C. perfringens* has been a main beneficiary.

That said, the illness caused by this bacteria is normally neither long-lasting nor particularly devastating. From within eight to twenty-two hours after ingesting the tainted food, the patient will suffer intense abdominal cramps and diarrhea. Usually, the whole episode will pass within a day.

There are, however, rare cases when a more virulent strain of the bacteria strikes. That causing gas gangrene is associated with infected wounds and quickly results in heart murmurs. Its designation comes from the fact that the bacteria releases CO_2 and hydrogen, "resulting in gas in the soft tissues and the emission of foul-smelling gas from the wound."[73] This disease is usually fatal, as is necrotic enteritis, which is induced by consuming large quantities of the bacteria. The enteritis kills by destroying intestinal cells and flooding the bloodstream. Although both of these *C. perfringens*-caused illnesses are rare, they are the ones those making biological weapons would be most interested in spreading.

There is no available treatment for these forms of food poisoning, which in the vast majority of cases run their course swiftly enough to necessitate little intervention, though their long-term consequences still need to be understood so as to be forestalled.

GLANDERS

Glanders is a bacterial disease that infects horses, donkeys, and mules and which is occasionally passed to humans. Cases of human infection are still found in Asia, Africa, the Middle East, and South America, but there has been only one incident of glanders in the United States in the past sixty-four years.

Interestingly, it is the equine aspects of the disease that have garnered the most attention from biological warriors. World War I is primarily known for the use of chemical weapons, such as mustard gas, but a pioneering effort in biowar was also carried out by the Austrians with the intention of weakening their Russian opponents. "Glanders was believed to have been spread deliberately...to infect large numbers of Russian horses and mules on the Eastern Front. This had an effect on troop and supply convoys as well as on artillery movements which were dependent on horses and mules."[74] The Germans, meanwhile, hatched a plot to infect horses bound for England with hopes that the disease would spread among herds in their British enemy's heartland.

The disease does spread quite readily between animals, but is less transmittable to human beings. In the past man has seldom been infected despite frequent and often close contact with infected animals.[75] When the disease does jump species, it is usually to infect veterinarians, those who care for animals, or slaughterhouse workers.

It can spread through inhalation or through cuts, and the disease can take four forms. It may manifest as *septicemic* (infecting the bloodstream). This form begins with fever, sweats, chest pain, tearing, and diarrhea, which may lead to rapid heartbeat and diseases of glands and liver. This form is quickly fatal. *Pulmonary* glanders begins with the same symptoms as the septicemic form, then may go on to bring on pneumonia and lesions in the lung. *Acute infection*, which occurs in the mouth or nose, is associated with "macopurulent, blood-streaked discharge from the nose," ulcerations on the skin and a rash similar to that found in smallpox.[76] The *chronic* form is characterized by abscesses in the arms and legs and enlargement of the lymph nodes. Recovery from this last form is possible, though it is also possible that it will transform into the septicemic form.

A number of traditional antibiotics, including sulfadiazine, doxycycline, rifampin, trimethoprim-sulfamethoxazole and ciprofloxacin have proven effective in combating glanders in experimental animal trials. However there have been so few cases of human infection, that it has been impossible to study treatments on them.

Let's look for a moment at that one United States case that was seen in the last sixty-odd years. It was written up in the *New England Journal of Medicine* by Arjun Srinivasan and others in an article that both details the case and concludes with some tersely worded, suggestive extrapolations.

The thirty-three-year-old man who came down with the disease in March 2000 was employed at the United States Army Medical Institute where for two years he had been studying the bacteria that produces glanders. He began experiencing fever and swollen glands, and treatment with a standard drug was ineffective. At this point, no diagnosis could be made. His disease progressed to fatigue, night sweats, and weight loss, but still his symptoms puzzled the doctors. He was admitted to Johns Hopkins, where tomography showed spleen and liver abscesses. Still, what was causing his problems was undetected as of yet.

(We bring your attention to Johns Hopkins, not because it is any less efficient at disease prevention than others, but because it is highly ironic that this is the same hospital where Dr. Bartlett brought his imaginary anthrax case, which also was incorrectly diagnosed all down the line.)

A tissue sample from the liver abscess as well as blood culture revealed the presence of the microbe behind glanders. Now treatment could proceed vigorously.

The good news is that antibiotics proved effective. First used were imipenem and doxycycline. Then, after two weeks, azithromycin was substituted for imipenem, and the patient was put on a six-week regimen. This seemed to have conquered the disease, and "one year later the patient remained in good health."[77]

Less reason for optimism is given by the length of time it took to learn what was wrong with the patient. "This case demonstrates," the authors write, "the difficulties that microbiology labs may have in recognizing potential agents of biological warfare. These microbes are rarely encountered and may be misidentified."[78] One wonders why the fact that the patient was working with glanders germs did not alert the doctors to what was going on, but it is possible, given the classified nature of this work, he didn't even tell his caretakers. This point is not illuminated in the journal article.

A second distressing point is also made. "This case may serve as a harbinger of the resurgence of nearly forgotten diseases such as glanders, plague, smallpox, and anthrax. Research on these disease is now being conducted in more laboratories."[79] This is yet another indication of how changing life patterns can play into the hands of the bad bugs.

Q FEVER *(Coxiella burnetti)*

The name "Q fever" derives from the fact that in Australia when the disease was first noticed, its cause could not be determined. It was dubbed "Query fever" to indicate that there was an ongoing query into its etiology.

Even now this disease is hard to pin down, presenting with a series of symptoms, such as fever, chills, cough, headache, weakness and chest pains, that are common to any number of diseases. There is nothing to distinguish it from a virus or an atypical pneumonia except that it is caused by a particular bacteria, *Coxiella burnetti*. This feature would make it an attractive biological warfare agent insofar as those first stricken by it would show no distinctive disease features, and so it would take a while before doctors traced the outbreak to its source in terrorism.

Balanced against this, though, are a number of minuses from the point of view of terrorists. For one, the fever is not transmitted from person to person, and so would not keep spreading beyond those who were initially infected. Moreover, the relatively mild symptoms only quite rarely develop into a serious disease. The illness lasts from a couple of days to a couple of weeks without serious or lingering effects.

The earlier reference to Australia, where Q fever was first sighted, might alert you to the fact that this disease is particularly spread to humans by contact with sheep. Australia has long been the prime sheep rancher for the world.

It can also be contracted via exposure to infected goats and cattle. The responsible bacteria "grows to especially high concentrations in placental tissues. Exposure to infected animals at parturition is an important risk factor for endemic disease."[80] The infection is passed through the air, with the victim inhaling the bacterial spore. The ability of this sporelike form to withstand heat and drying and to survive on inanimate surfaces allows the organisms to persist in the environment for weeks or months after infected animals have vacated an area and to be transported by the wind to disseminate the infections at sites miles distant from the source.

Treatments of acute Q fever shorten the course of the disease and prevent the disease from manifesting when administered during the incubation period, which is from two days to two weeks. Tetracyclines remain the mainstay of traditional therapy for the acute form. Macrolide antibiotics, such as erythromycin and azithromycin, are also effective. Quinolones, chloramphenicol and trimethoprim-sulphamethoxazole have also been used to treat Q fever, but clinical experience with these drugs is limited.

RICIN TOXIN FROM RICINUS COMMUNIS (castor beans)

As already noted, biowarfare agents do not only include bacteria or viruses that have suffered militarization but also involve more inactive elements derived from living sources, such as the plant toxin ricin.

Like glanders, the ricin toxin has great historical interest as one of the earliest biological derivatives put to use for lethal purposes. During World War II, the Japanese performed horrific experiments on prisoners of war to assess the effects of different dosages of this toxin. Contemporaneously, the United States was trying to gauge the toxin's killing power, using animals as ricin's victims.

More notoriously, during the Cold War, ricin toxin was employed in a notably successful assassination attempt. As is described in *No Fire, No Thunder*, the Bulgarian Communist government wanted to eliminate two dissident exiles. "Georgi Markov, an exile resident in London, was killed in September 1978 by a pellet containing ricin which had been shot into his leg."[81] An attack on another exile, Vladimir Kostov, failed because the pellet was slowed by his thick winter clothing and didn't penetrate to the skin.

This toxin was one of the first developed by governments interested in biological warfare because of its ready availability and ease of manufacture. The poison is extracted from the bean of the castor plant, the same bean from which castor oil is produced. The toxin makes up a small percentage of the waste products from manufacture of the oil. Where other potential agents of biological war would have to be obtained through lab culture of germs or the extraction of the sickness-dealing agent from plants or animals, the enterprising terrorist could get ahold of ricin toxin by raiding and sifting through the refuse from a castor oil production facility. This has made it attractive.

On the down side, from a biowarfare purveyor's view, is the fact that

> it is of marginal toxicity [in terms of the need for a large amount to be inhaled for it to have a devastating effect]…in comparison to toxins such as botulism…so an enemy would have to produce it in larger quantities to cover a significant area on the battlefield.[82]

A person could be exposed to the toxin in a number of ways, including in food or drink or through an aerosol. Since it is rarely contacted naturally, except through eating castor beans, which are not a foodstuff, most study of the effect of the toxin has looked at how it would strike through inhalation—the most likely way bioterrorists would disseminate it. Within four to eight hours after breathing in the toxin, a patient would be beset by fever, a tightness in the chest, cough, joint pain, nausea, and labored breathing. Presumably, death would occur through the destruction of bodily tissues, which would be killed by ricin's blockages of the body's synthesis of proteins. (No human deaths have been described by scientists, so estimates on the course of a fatal termination are based on animal models.) If, on the other hand, the dosage has not been sufficient to cause death, the onset of profuse sweating indicates one has begin to recover.

There is no treatment for poisoning by ricin toxin at present, though various vaccines are being developed.

STAPHYLOCOCCAL ENTEROTOXIN TYPE B (SEB)

Staphylococcus enterotoxin type B (SEB) is produced by *Staphylococcus aureus* bacteria. SEB is excreted as waste material by the bacteria and, if the germ has found its way into a human, the toxin plays havoc with the intestines.

Today, SEB is regularly contracted through food poisoning. We've already noted that incidences of this poisoning in the United States have increased with changes in eating habits, and recent cases of *S. aureus* poisoning reflect this alteration. For example, a case occurred in sixteen elementary schools in Texas when 1,364 kids were taken sick after eating chicken salad. Investigation showed that to prepare this meal the chicken had been boiled for three hours, then deboned and cooled to room temperature by fans. "Contamination of the chicken probably occurred when it was deboned. The chicken was not cooled rapidly enough because it was stored in twelve-inch-deep layers."[83] The still warm under-chicken, which probably received the germ from an infected kitchen hand, was the breeding ground for the bacteria.

In the section on *Clostridium perfringens,* we discussed such cases, which reflect on the special hazards of mass producing meals, we also noted Schlosser's opinion that the real villain in most food poisoning incidents were the companies that supplied the meal makers. An illustrative case from 1989 documents the different kind of problems that can occur when the food comes tainted to the restaurant.

On February 13, in Starkville, Mississippi, twenty-two people got sick after eating in a university cafeteria. Nine entered hospitals. On investigating the outbreak, "no deficiencies in food handling were found."[84] The culprit was the canned mushrooms "served with omelets and hamburgers." A second flare-up took place fifteen days later, this time in a Queens, New York, hospital cafeteria. After eating mushrooms from the salad bar, forty-eight people became sick. A month and a half later, twelve diners got sick in McKeesport, Pennsylvania, from consuming *staphylococcus*-laced mushrooms on their pizzas or in parmigiana sauce at a popular restaurant. Then, a few days later, on April 22, twenty people who had eaten take-out pizza in Philipsburg, Pennsylvania, were sickened the same way from the same comestible.

The FDA doesn't make clear whether all these canned mushrooms were coming from the same company, all this is what the report suggests. Yet, at the same time, one would hope the erring mushrooms would have been recalled by the time of the fourth eruption, which was two months after the first.

This is where *Fast Food Nation* is so sobering. Although author Schlosser is not concerned with mushrooms, but meat, he does paint a distressing picture of how lax government oversight agencies can be when it comes to policing food production.

In January 1993, it might be recalled, seven hundred people in four states were sickened by *E. coli* infection passed to them through hamburgers purchased at Jack in the Box. Four people died from the infection. After this scandal, there was some reform in government meat inspection, which had been increasingly weakened under the deregulation cowboys, Reagan and Bush. These presidents, "cut spending on public health measures and staffed the United States Department of Agriculture with officials far more interested in government deregulation than in food safety."[85] Reagan's secretary of agriculture, for instance, was in the pig business; while the man he picked to run the USDA's inspection service was vice-president of the National Cattlemen's Association. They oversaw the introduction of a new program, which "was designed to reduce the presence of federal inspectors in the nation's slaughterhouses, allowing company employees to assume most of the food safety tasks."[86]

The outcry over the Jack in the Box poisonings, which were due to the presence of *E. coli* in batches of meat from Vons Co. meat processors, changed things, but just a little. President Clinton promised to clean up the industry, but, like his much-vaunted promise of healthcare reform, this program was derailed by industry and Republican militant resistance. Schlosser points out, by the way, that Speaker of the House Newt Gingrich, who led the charge against Clinton on this and other policies, "received more money from the restaurant industry than any other representative."[87] Like the meat industry executives that filled Reagan and Bush administration posts, the current crop of pro-industry federal legislators (whose campaign chests overflow with contributions from meatpackers) have "spent a great deal of effort in denying the federal government any authority to recall contaminated meat or impose civil fines on firms that knowingly ship contaminated products."[88] So, the industry has kept things the way it likes them.

> Under current law, the USDA cannot demand a recall [when it finds contaminated meat on the market]. It can only consult with a company that has shipped bad meat and suggest that it withdraw the meat from interstate commerce.... Once a company has decided to voluntarily to pull contaminated meat from the market, it is under no legal obligation to inform the public—or even state health officials—that a recall is taking place.[89]

Thus, in line with the last point, when Nevada Jack in the Boxes started sending back the meat patties that were causing hundreds of poisonings, they didn't tell the state what was going on. State officials figured it out "when people noticed trucks pulling up to Jack in the Box restaurants in Las Vegas and removing the meat."[90] If all this isn't enough to indicate how supine the federal inspection agencies are when it comes to keeping our food safe, note further that if a producer whose meat is poisoning consumers *decides* to recall that product, it is up to the producer to decide how much is to be taken back and, until recently, the government allowed the affected company to *help write the USDA press release* about the recalls!

It's hardly a pretty picture. Right when surveillance of food becomes particularly important, with more people making a switch over to fast and institutional food, government watchdogs are snoozing. We would need the three-headed Cerberus to really keep an eye on these lax meatpackers, but instead we get a government canine as feeble as Ulysses' pet. (The dog waited ten years for his master's return, then dropped dead on first seeing him.)

All said, SEB is hardly the worst of the toxins that are commonly ingested from food. When one eats food contaminated with staphylococcal enterotoxin type B, a few hours later there is nausea, vomiting and non-bloody diarrhea. Usually the situation resolves itself within twelve to twenty-four hours. Many cases are so mild that they are not recognized as due to food poisoning. There is no treatment that would alleviate the effect of the poison.

It is thought that if this toxin is made use of for chemical warfare purposes it will be manufactured as an aerosol. If a person is exposed to inhalational SEB, the symptoms would be fever, chills, headache, muscle pain, and coughing. The fever would last two to five days; while the cough would continue for a month. All these prognoses are, of course, suppositional since there have not yet been cases of inhalational SEB.

SEB, like the just-mentioned ricin toxin, has played a role in the history of biological warfare. At the time of the Cuban Missile Crisis, when President Kennedy faced down Cuba, telling the Caribbean country it must remove its Soviet-supplied rockets or face invasion, biological weapons were prepared in case the worst came to pass. Fort Detrick developed a special "cocktail," which included the germs that produce Q fever, Venezuelan equine encephalitis along with staphylococcal enterotoxin type B. These were made into a liquid that could be sprayed on the unsuspecting and produced to the tune of thousands of gallons.

> [According to the military plan] exposure to the agents would debilitate Cubans within a few hours and the incapacitation would last up to three weeks. Jets would tank up at Pine Bluff's airfield, fly to Cuba, and spray the concoction over key towns, ports, and military bases.[91]

Fortunately for everyone, this payload was never delivered, since it would have produced untold suffering as well as an estimated 70,000 deaths.

This plan also indicates the potential usefulness of the less devastating biological warfare agents. There may be situations, such as the Cuban one, in which what is wanted is the temporary weakening, not the elimination, of enemy forces. Then, something far short of the more potent germs will be desirable. Thus it is that all countries capable of developing this form of bioweaponry have simultaneously tried to perfect different agents so as to have in their quivers arrows with all types of heads.

CATEGORY C

The diseases that fall under this heading are ones that do not now seem to pose much risk of being wielded by terrorists either because they are not readily available or creatable or do not have a potential, if weaponized, for having much of an impact on the health of those who contract the illness. However, as our book's opening discussion of multi-drug resistant tuberculosis has suggested, such germs do not need the sponsorship of governments or terrorist cells in order to attack populations.

MULTI-DRUG-RESISTANT TUBERCULOSIS (MDR-TB)

We began this book by describing the rise of a new strain of tuberculosis that eluded the power of most antibiotics. Later, we highlighted that such strains were produced when a patient failed to follow his or her drug regimen, lapsing in the taking of medication as soon as the manifest symptoms of the disease disappeared. There is no need to excessively belabor this point, although it is worth saying that, contrary to popular prejudice, the new forms of TB are not exclusive to the poorer sides of big Eastern cities.

Garrett details a case that occurred in Davidson County, North Carolina. A thirty-two-year-old man died of MDR-TB in April 1984. In a follow-up, the CDC tested his family and acquaintances for the disease. They found that his neighbor, the neighbor's girlfriend, his brother (who lived in another state), and a drinking buddy all tested positive for multi-drug resistant tuberculosis. All had been under treatment for the disease at one time or another. The neighbor seemed to have been the first developer of the strain since he had TB on and off for six years. He was an alcoholic, and he and the others "spent hours drinking together in a local bar. Because the anti-tuberculosis drugs could not be tolerated with alcohol, the individuals failed to follow medication instructions."[92] All but the girlfriend died of TB.

If one wanted to second guess Garrett, one could say (erroneously) that her obvious reason for delving into this case is to indicate that self-indulgent behavior, which gives a green light to newly emerging germs, is found everywhere, from the great metropolises to the rural South. However, her main interest in presenting this anecdote is to discuss problems in the United

States health system, not this particular group of heavy imbibers. After saying a few words about the tuberculosis in general, we will come back to a discussion of this incident, which will return us to one of our grand themes, the relation between collective and personal responsibility.

Just as smallpox is so named because of pock marks that appear on a sufferer's face and bubonic plague given its denomination due to the presence of "buboes" (the old name for swollen glands), so the word "tuberculosis" derives from the patient's "tubercles," which are a series of small round swellings, which are found on the lungs and other parts of the body.

TB is produced by infection with the bacteria, whose name is self-explanatory, *Mycobacterium tuberculosis*. The disease is contagious, spread between people by particles suspended in the breath or coughs of an infected person. This does not mean, however, that the disease is easily contracted. One has to have prolonged contact with a person with TB in order to come down with the illness. Further, a robust immune system can fight off the disease, as has been shown by people that are healthy and who were never apparently infected, but who reveal healed tubercle scars on X-rays, indicating that they were touched by the bacteria at one time.

Since the disease is generally spread through the air, primary infection will normally occur in the lungs, although the bacteria can take root in any portion of the body.

In the first stages of the disease, the TB patient has fevers, a weight loss and lessened strength. If the disease is allowed to progress, it will result in sneezing, breathing difficulties, and the coughing up of blood. Death is the final result if the patient does not respond to treatment.

Until recently, patients did respond to protracted bed rest in combination with months of administration of such drugs as streptomycin, isoniazid, seromycin, and viomycin. If the TB reaches an advanced form, it is necessary to excise part of the infected lung.[93]

Recently, as we have seen, emerging forms of tuberculosis are less pliant. This is not only because, since they are facing a disease that is making a comeback, clinics may not be conversant with the optimum treatments. Even the best equipped health centers are failing to make much headway against MRD-TBs. Garrett talked to Dr. Michael Iseman, chief TB physician at the National Jewish Center for Immunology and Respiratory Medicine in Denver. "Iseman announced that even in his hands, in the best TB treatment center in the entire world, MDR-TB was extremely lethal."[94] Touching on the fate of 171 patients with multi-drug resistant tuberculosis under his charge, he noted that more than one third "showed no response whatsoever to treatment [after the normally used drugs failed], with remaining theoretically effective drugs."[95] Half of this 171 never recovered, either dying or living on with reduced capability due to the lingering disease.

Moreover, this situation is not likely to change for the better in the short run, since there are no new drugs or therapies in the medical pipeline. In the early 1990s, the National Institute for Allergy and Infectious Diseases (NIAID) began prioritizing TB studies again, but this was after they had been in abeyance for decades. As Dr. Barry Bloom from WHO commented, "Essentially everything that is known about tuberculosis was figured out before 1948, when antibiotics came into use. And virtually all research stopped after that. Dead stop."[96]

But let's get back to our story about North Carolina. Garrett's conclusion after explaining how the patients were reluctant to follow their doctor's prescriptions, is this: "Nobody from the city, county, or state public health systems took steps at any time between 1978 to 1985 to track the recalcitrant patients or force medication compliance."[97] Moreover, this finding is no anomaly in terms of United States healthcare. As Harvard medical economist Christopher Murray found in a comparative study of medical performance around the world, "No nation's TB control system did a poorer job than did that of the United States in identifying tuberculosis cases, successfully treating those cases, and keeping track of their outcome and possible contacts."[98] A prime reason for the unexpected pitifulness of the United States effort is that unlike those countries with high success rates in handling this illness, countries such as Nicaragua, Tanzania, and Mozambique, we do not devote considerable manpower to keeping tabs on patients.

Although in 1992 the New York City Department of Health, working with the CDC, reversed the poor figures it was recording in obtaining compliance to drug regimens and curing TB by instituting follow-up programs whereby TB sufferers would be taken in hand by newly trained nonprofessionals, there are two broader United States social patterns that work against such reversals.

For one, the medical infrastructure is resolutely high end. That is to say, its emphasis has long been on complicated, expensive surgeries and treatments, such as putting in artificial hearts, which have been backed by sophisticated tests, such as the PCR examination, which will identify individual proteins in blood. These procedures are all capital intensive. They rely on advanced technology and highly trained operatives. What the Third World countries that achieved extraordinary victories over TB had to offer was low-end, labor-intensive care. They were lacking in all the advanced equipment available in Western hospitals, but they did have plenty of *personnel*, health workers who had the time to keep watch on TB sufferers, visiting their homes frequently, and accompanying them to the clinic. It would seem, then, that certain types of illness are best confronted by supportive human intervention. To face down multi-drug-resistant tuberculosis in particular, our health care must, as it did in New York City, be ready for a retooling of outlooks and approaches.

Difficult as such a changeover would be, Garrett implies there is an even more deep-lying problem facing our public health system. An important reason behind the original lack of patient compliance with both the North Carolina and New York City medical dictates is that *there was no continuum between doctors and patients*. We have already remarked on the two-tiered health care now in place in our nation. Those without health care or resources lack personal physicians and rely on emergency rooms for treatment. They are not able to put a face on those treating them, in the sense that they do not have time or consistent contact with specific medical workers to build a relationship. Moreover, as Garrett clarifies, most of the MDR-TB patients are single men from the bottom rungs of the economy, circulating through homeless shelters and prisons. They are outcasts, alienated from mainstream society. Those in this position are the least likely to do what professionals tell them is best for their health, since their connection to professionals, from prison guards to shelter workers, has probably been largely unfriendly. Outside of making medical care freely available to all, it would seem there is not much to be done about this aspect of the situation. But, seeing as the resistant TB that is most prominent in this group has spread to social workers, doctors, nurses, and guards, it would seem no part of society will stand protected from the new TB unless we find a way to give everyone some small stake in everyone else's well being. How and whether this can be done will be discussed later. For now, let us just reiterate the meaning of Garrett's example.

As she makes clear, what riles her is not the fecklessness of those TB-infected drinkers in North Carolina so much as the careless and callous health care system that didn't keep tabs on them. This is not to say that they should not be held responsible for their own downfall, but to add that responsibility has to be shared. *Health is a possession of a community*.

NIPAH VIRUS

We've seen throughout these presentations that at the same time as humans have been able to eliminate some diseases, such as smallpox, that have long harried civilization; new diseases have come forward. In 1953, the first cases of Argentine hemorrhagic fever appeared, while in 1969 Lassa fever was introduced. Ebola virus is of even more recent vintage, originally surfacing in 1976. The late comer of all the new diseases, though, is Nipah virus, which was first seen in 1998. In outbreaks that year and the next, it killed 106 people in Singapore and Malaysia.

Even more unsettling was a report in *Science* that said this and another relatively new virus, Hendra virus, "are representative of a new genus within the family Paramyxoviridae."[99] The reason the authors feel a new classification is necessary is "like Hendra virus, Nipah virus is unusual among the paramyxoviridae in its ability to infect and cause potentially fatal disease in a number of host species, including humans."[100]

It is believed that the animal reservoir for the illness is a fruit bat that is found in Australia, the Philippines, Indonesia, Malaysia, and smaller Pacific islands. In the recent occurrences, it was passed to humans through contact with pigs. The CDC reports, "Eight-six percent of case-patients reported touching or handling pigs before onset of illness.... [Further] human-to-human transmission of Nipah virus has not been encountered."[101] The Far Eastern eruption of the disease quickly came to end when the pigs who were carrying the disease were eliminated (a million were killed), the transportation of the animals from one area to another was halted, and government surveillance was established to detect new cases among the livestock.

Once a person is infected with the virus, it takes between four and eighteen days before the symptoms begin to manifest. A mild case will appear as a flu, while a serious case will begin with flu-like symptoms, such as fever and aches and pains. The sickness may then lead to inflammation of the brain, disorientation, convulsions, and coma.

As with many of the diseases we have been discussing, there is no treatment that can counteract the virus, but supportive care and bed rest should palliate the condition to some extent. According to WHO, "There is some evidence that early treatment with the antiviral drug, ribavirin, can reduce both the duration of feverish illness and the severity of the disease."[102] However, all attempts to find treatments to stave off or limit the effectiveness of the virus are still in an experimental stage.

TICKBORNE ENCEPHALITIS VIRUS (Powassan or POW virus)

Bacteria and viruses come in different strains. Tickborne viral encephalitis, for example, is related to three other tickborne encephalitic viruses that are exclusive to the Eastern hemisphere. These range in severity from the Louping-ill, which seldom strikes humans and causes an uncomplicated flu-like disease, to Russian spring-summer encephalitis, which is characterized by violent headache, high fever, and nausea, leading in the worst cases to coma and death.[103]

Tickborne viral encephalitis (also known as Powassan encephalitis) had not been seen in the United States since 1994 when a handful of new cases appeared from 1999 to 2001. One case described by *JAMA* was that of a seventy-year-old man from Maine, who reported to the hospital with muscle weakness, diarrhea, and anorexia. He suffered what appeared to be a stroke, and three months after onset "he remains in the facility and is unable to move his left arm or leg."[104] An investigation of the cause of his illness, which was identified as Powassan virus, seemed to indicate a tick-bite. His property was covered with overgrown bushes, disused lumber, and leaves, ideal hiding places for tick-infected rodents, and over the two weeks previous to his sickness, he had been working on a boat, lying on his back in the yard.

A second case was that of a fifty-three-year-old woman, also from Maine, who came into the hospital with a high fever, weakness, and visual impairment. After two months in rehabilitation, she was released, but nine months later, she still suffered from trouble seeing. Her infection seemed to have come about when she was cleaning out some squirrels nests at her vacation home. *MMWR* remarks that the ticks that harbor this virus, unlike those that are a reservoir for Lyme disease and which often are found on vegetation, tend to live near animal burrows and nests when they are not actually on a mammal. Neither of these stricken people, by the way, remembered being bitten by ticks, but, the report notes, "Few infected people recalled tick bites because these tick bites are small and can be easily missed."[105]

Illness brought on by the ticks begins with high fever, muscle aches and pains, and diarrhea. It can lead to brain inflammation and, in 10 to 15 percent of cases, death.

There is no viable treatment or vaccine against the disease, and supportive care is the most that can be given to victims. The only thing to do is to ward off the disease in the first place by wearing protective clothing, leaving no exposed skin, staying away from brush and cleaning it from one's property, using insect repellents, and checking pets so that they don't transport ticks into the home.

YELLOW FEVER

If Ebola virus appears to the general public a thing to be feared, then yellow fever probably is considered a disease that has largely vanished from the earth.

In the 1940s, a Hollywood film was made celebrating the exploits of Dr. Walter Reed. Reed, seeing that the French gave up on an attempt to dig the

Panama Canal because so many of their workers were prostrated by yellow fever, set out to tame the disease. In 1901, he and Cuban doctor Carlos Finley determined the disease was being spread by a particular mosquito that laid eggs in clear water, such as that kept by people in cisterns. Simply covering these potential birthing places would go a long way to reducing disease occurrence. Taking a cue from these discoveries, Major William Gorgas of the United States Army set out to eradicate the disease in Havana. "The campaign was so successful that within several months yellow fever had almost disappeared from the city. [Then] in 1905 Gorgas was sent to Panama to combat yellow fever there."[106]

In 1927, a vaccine was developed. At this point, the first official world campaign to eliminate a disease was undertaken, and efforts went forward to completely stamp out the offensive *A. aegypti* mosquito.

The project bogged down shortly thereafter, however, when it was discovered that there were two forms of the disease, one, the urban form, harbored by *aegypti* and, the other, the jungle version, with a reservoir in monkey populations from which it passed to various mosquito species. While the first discovered form could be near eliminated by killing mosquitoes, "the jungle form could not be eliminated without vaccinating all wild monkeys in Africa and South America, a clearly impossible task."[107] Moreover, even the will to

> persist in the struggle against the urban form, which is the one that causes the most cases, seems lacking. As Garrett documents, proposals floated in the early 1970s that would have the United States government acting to wipe out the *aegypti* mosquito were shot down by those who felt it would be too expensive, especially given that many American property owners would object to spraying on their land and would have to be taken to court to enforce control measures.[108]

Unfortunately, the public is more likely to remember the heroic story about Walter Reed than know about the subsequent loss of hope in permanently eliminating the disease. After all, no Hollywood film was made about the failure of the effort.

The disease causes either a mild or severe illness. In its milder version, the sufferer has merely a mild fever and headache. The stronger version begins with headache, back pain, nausea and vomiting. The name of the disease comes from the jaundice that appears on about the fourth day. There is then often internal hemorrhaging. In the worst cases, the patient falls into coma and dies somewhere between the sixth and ninth day.

There is no treatment to reverse the effects of the disease, and this is why authorities caution travelers to become immunized before traveling to places where the disease is endemic.

CRITIQUE OF GARRETT

Context and Community

———

W e have borrowed rather freely from the works of Laurie Garrett in con-
structing the first part of this examination. Not only does she, in her
two definitive books, offer a wealth of information on the rise of new diseases and the reappearance of once-moribund ones, but she is a empathetic
and colorful travel writer, as it were, giving illuminating sketches of different
parts of the world that have hosted disease outbreaks, so that the reader
feels part of the scene and understands the milieu. Further, her grand thesis,
which is that the danger of new disease outbreaks is magnified in the United
States by the remiss treatment of public health, is a theme with which we
heartily concur.

Yet, there are two places where, as I see it, she underplays materials that
I believe should be given more prominence. Sometimes she draws back before laying out the complete picture. Sometimes, she doesn't follow through
on her deepest insights by connecting them up to her basal theme. The first
happens in terms of context, the second in relation to the part the overall
community must take in promoting public health.

The broader story is not given, for instance, when she outlines the reasons for the failure of yellow fever mosquito elimination campaign. The way
American political exigencies clouded the issue is clear, but not the reason
diseases such as yellow fever were targeted in the first place, over other can-
didate illnesses.

———

The project began with high hopes. "Public health officials were confident the insect could be wiped out of the Americas by the mid-1960s."[109] As we saw, these hopes were ill-founded because of the number of animal reservoirs and the half-hearted commitment of the government. Yet, if one looked deeper, it would become evident that Western medicine had long divided tropical diseases into two categories, ones that arose from poor sanitation and other deficit living conditions and ones that could spread between natives and Europeans. Only the latter were of interest.

Doyal and Pennell argue that Westerners' interest in controlling yellow fever, malaria, and sleeping sickness, all insect-vector diseases, needs to be understood in light of colonialism. Western medical service sectors that were created in the tropical regions the late nineteenth century had an overwhelming interest in the health of European colonial troops and masters. Native workers in the mines and plantations were so plentiful as to be expendable. It was easier to replace them than to provide healthcare.

Since the natives who were uprooted and brought to the cities tended to get sick, the first concern of Western doctors was to keep their patients away from the colonized. "There was an overwhelming fear of contagion [passed from the colonized] among the ruling class, and in the colonial context the response was physically to exclude the agents of infection by legally enforcing a system of racial segregation."[110] Certain sections of the Third World cities were designated for Whites only, while others were the domain of the country's original inhabitants. This saved on funding, since "this arrangement lent itself to the selective introduction of amenities [such as clean water, garbage disposal, and sewage systems] for whites."[111] At the same time, natives were condemned to endemic disease in that "there was a systematic denial of public health provisions to the non-white population."[112]

Looking at the situation in East Africa, Doyal and Pennell note that cruel as such social arrangements may seem, they worked quite well for the generality of diseases, but there were two that couldn't be so easily controlled.

> Most of the diseases which were becoming [in the late nineteenth century] endemic in east Africa were of little consequence to Europeans, because they were usually contracted directly through exposure to bad living conditions. There were, however, two important exceptions—malaria and sleeping sickness.... Their insect vectors showed little racial discrimination.... Because these two diseases impinged so directly on metropolitan interests, attempts to

control them provided the main focus for colonial medical
activity and absorbed a large proportion of limited health
resources in the region. This overriding concern with
malaria and sleeping sickness was also reflected at the international level among the various precursors of the World
Health Organization.[113]

The more recent battle against yellow fever in Latin and South America,
though less blatantly colonialist, appears to stem from a similar desire to
protect the interests of Westerners rather than aid indigenous people in the
poorer lands. Countries that were being fitted out as major trading partners
for Western businesses were where the eradication campaigns were di-
rected. "While campaigns were strongly focused on Asia and Latin America,
virtually nothing was attempted in sub-Saharan Africa which at that time
was becoming increasingly marginal within the international economy."[114]

A second weakness of emphasis appears in how the lessons of such
episodes as that of eradication of the Hanta virus outbreak in the South-
western United States are not woven into her grand theme. Although that
episode made it loud and clear that true public health is born when the
community and medical workers combine their efforts, engaging in authen-
tic give and take, when it comes to prescriptions for the future, Garrett con-
centrates on better funding and staffing of public health services. She does
not underline how improved public health is dependent on the full enroll-
ment of the community in health efforts, though there is more than enough
material in her exposition to indicate the strength of such alliances and the
disasters that occur when this connection is let lapse.

Studies of colonial Africa are rife with stories of how the colonial masters, secure in their sense of superiority, interfered with native disease prevention practices and suffered the consequences.

To mention only one such circumstance, let us refer to attempts to curtail sleeping sickness by the British rulers of nineteenth-century East Africa.
In the nineteenth century, African herdsmen kept substantial amounts of
cattle, and to do so, they had to minimize the impingement of tsetse flies,
who spread sleeping sickness to the cows. "The tsetse were known to thrive
in dense brush inhabited by an abundance of wild animals. Thus, African
pastoralists…employed a wide range of preventive measures such as bush
clearing and game control."[115]

The ability to carry out these public health practices ended after the European invasion, which seriously reduced manpower in the villages. For one,

many natives were killed in the attempt to resist European usurpations. Second, once colonial governments took charge men were forced to move out of the villages into work camps. The coercion behind this displacement was generally the imposition of monetary taxes onto a barter economy. Only through paid work was it possible to accrue money to pay off the taxes, so most able-bodied males had to hire on at plantations or sites of extractive industries. Women stayed behind to maintain the land, but they were insufficient in numbers to keep cutting back the bush and killing excessive animals. Nor could the remaining tribespeople manage to care for large herds of grazing stock, which had been useful in trimming back vegetation.

The disease began killing not only the remnants of cattle herds but also the villagers. The colonialist administrators' approaches to the situation were counterproductive. In Tanganyika, "the British, for example, ordered the mass evacuation of Africans from the advancing tsetse fly belts and their resettlement in new 'concentrations.'"[116] Thus, the depredations of the tsetse were tacitly accepted as the ground was given over to them. The result was that the retreat of the natives meant the tsetse could extend their range, which went from about one third of the country in 1913 to fully three quarters of the country by 1948.

We don't want to multiply bad examples. It is more important to stress the positive idea that public health is tied to community empowerment. Let's move beyond a critique of Garrett to study a case history that will investigate the confluence of public health and a city's people during a time of epidemic. We will show that when a public is fully involved in fighting in a health crisis, it may have to overturn the government, even, as we will see, the government of the United States, to ensure survival.

YELLOW FEVER

AND COMMUNITY HEALTH

Philadelphia 1793

___

In late July 1793 a Philadelphia doctor recognized a case of yellow fever. Within three months the fever had killed 5,000 of the city's 51,000 inhabitants and driven an additional 17,000 to flight. Those who left were those who could afford to. The poor and public spirited stayed in place. Included among the decampers were the governor, President Washington, and other members of the federal government. Philadelphia was the nation's temporary capital, since Washington, D.C., was still under construction.

"By early September so many members of established institutions—from the presidency of the United States on down—had either died or fled the city that 'government of every kind was almost wholly vacated.'"[117] According to historian Sally Griffith, with government in abeyance; most civic institutions, such as churches, reading rooms, and coffee houses, closed for fear of contagion; essential services, such as burying the dead, decayed; and human contact itself ground to a halt, since everyone barricaded themselves in their houses. Griffith puts it that "the city descended into anarchy."[118] This does not mean there was looting or law breaking; but that the normal bonds of human society did not hold. Wives would abandon husbands, children would leave their parents, all in a mad fear of infection.

After reaching this nadir of human compassion, city life was reignited when a voluntary government was created. On September 10, the mayor, one of the last remaining elected officials, called a meeting, open to all comers, from which he hoped to recruit citizens to take charge of nonoperational civic functions. From this assembly emerged a committee of ten, and later twenty-six, who self assigned themselves such jobs as directing the fever hospital at Bush Hill (itself an abandoned mansion pressed into service in the emergency), distributing aid, transporting the sick to the hospital and the dead away from it, and minding the numerous orphans.

Meanwhile, the small Black community of something over three thousand souls began to play a decisive role. At the time, it was believed Blacks were immune to yellow fever. Although this was not true, the observation may have had some factual grounding in that many Blacks had come from Africa or the West Indies where they might have been exposed to the disease and developed immunity. Feeling that Blacks were not liable to catch the fever, the improvised government "appealed to Jones [pastor of St. Thomas Church], Allen [Bishop of the African Methodist Episcopal Church], and other leaders of Philadelphia's free Black community to aid in the relief effort."[119] Blacks took up jobs nursing, patrolling the streets, checking abandoned property, transporting, grave digging, and even doctoring. The liberal physician Benjamin Rush (famous as signer of the Declaration of Independence) was a principled egalitarian, who said his methods of treating the fever could "be practiced by anyone with little formal training. Putting his beliefs into practice, he trained a group of free Blacks as itinerant bleeders during the epidemic."[120] In sum, "these humblest of Philadelphians, many recently slaves, helped administer what was effectively the government of the city."[121]

The ruling committee itself was largely staffed by the Jeffersonian faction of Philadelphia's middle class. At the time, the country was torn between the views of Treasury Secretary Alexander Hamilton, who feared mob rule and lawlessness, and those of Thomas Jefferson, who feared authoritarianism and the over-extension of the government's power. (Around these men would soon crystallize our country's first political parties, with the Hamiltonians becoming Federalists and the Jeffersonians becoming Republicans.) As Martin Pernick reports, the epidemic quickly became politicized, with each nascent group tending to espouse a party line on disease causation (believing either it was endemic or imported by immigrant carriers) and treatment methods. Significantly, it was the Republican faction which remained in town to man the ramparts, while Federalists generally took to their heels. By default, then, the temporary administration was one imbued with democratic principles.[122]

If we take this tale as representative, we can fashion some startling generalizations about disease, the government, and the citizenry.

As we saw, the state collapsed under the pressure of a medical crisis. The whole society, rather than disintegrating in turn, provided a more flexible civic structure, which was better able to cope with the new circumstances. Let's not call this new structure a "state" proper, but rather a "default proto state" (DPS), for reasons that will be clarified below. This surface zone differed from the previous institutions in four ways, namely:

■ It opened the consultative and executive functions of the government to excluded groups, such as to African-Americans, something unthinkable in less desperate situations.

■ It set aside normal procedures for the handling of civic administration, while, at the same time, replacing people's core motivations for wanting to work in such administration. More simply put, institutionalized methods for hiring people to run city services were dropped in favor of voluntarism and ad-hoc usages. People elected themselves to jobs, which jobs were carried out as they saw fit. This linked to a loss of the typical careerist motivations that formerly propelled people to work in the city government. The participants in the improvised government were not paid, nor were most advancing their careers, since few but the mayor would remain in politics once the crisis passed. Moreover, by taking these jobs, they thought they greatly increased their chances of death, since all believed the fever was contagious. Many died in the traces.

■ Moreover, it was not simply that people took up work that was congenial to them because they were already trained for it, as were, for example, the Caribbean immigrant doctors who volunteered at the Bush Hill facility. As we saw in the case of Rush's training of physicians, in some instances, there was an erasure of the line separating amateurs and professionals, as befitted the radical democracy espoused by the Republicans.

■ Lastly, in a point not brought up heretofore, there were *daily* meetings at which the committee would comment on difficulties and keep everyone updated. This practices, like the others mentioned, served to make the DPS more responsive to the immediate dimensions of the world, both because it was constantly surveying the ongoing events and because it was drawing more widely on resources available within its society, ones hitherto untapped because of prejudice, exclusionary professional criteria, and so on.

Once the three-month reign of the plague ended, the former governors trickled back into town and resumed their posts. In fact, as Pernick reports, the few who ran for office in the next election against those who had for-saken their posts, did not profit from their self-sacrifice. They were not voted in, which is not surprising in that many of the voters had themselves de-camped when the going got rough.[123]

This is why we call interim executive committee a surface phenomenon. Once the crisis past, the deep organizational structures of the government, which had been left intact, resumed operation. We might conclude the DPS was superficial, contingent, and of little impact. However, another way to view this is to say, that as long as the foundational structures of the society, such as the legality of slavery, the codification of limited manhood suffrage, and such like, were in place, any change that violated these parameters would not be sustainable. The most that could occur, in the sense of state forms that violated the general tenor of the social arrangement, would be an inscription on the surface of society that suggested directions in which the core might later evolve.

We can relate this to the concept of the TAZ (temporary autonomous zone) discussed in our work on AIDS.[124] Hakim Bey, who introduces this idea, wonders aloud if, in a rigidified, anomic society such as ours, it is still possible to achieve a sense of a better world." He asks, "Are we who live in the present doomed to never experience autonomy, never to stand for one mo-ment on a bit of land ruled only by freedom?"[125] He answers that a space of freedom can be created by engaging in disruptive but lyrical activities which briefly interrupt the organized rays of commerce and consumerism. (A good example would be the actions carried out in London by Free the Streets, such as when they blocked a major highway for hours for an illegal party.)

The Default Proto State, by contrast, is not the product of planning, but arises unintendedly when a particular society is about to capsize, as when Philadelphia was descending into anarchy. It is true that the righting meth-ods that emerged to keep the city afloat did have utopic elements, as did the TAZ, but where, dimensionally, the temporary zone created a pocket of mo-mentary resistance, the proto state refaced the whole governing operation. Like the TAZ, though, the proto state is limited in time, being in force only until the heavy pulse of the inequalitarian society begins beating again.

Be that as it may, our central ideas can be put in the form of two facts and a supposition.

FACT ONE: Under the onslaught of devastating epidemic, the public health system, along with the city government of which is was a part, stopped working.

FACT TWO: All the things that needed to be done to save Philadelphia were taken over by self-enlisted citizens who created from scratch or redesigned administrative services.

SUPPOSITION: This signalizes that critical health situations can best be dealt with by enlisting the public as co-creators with the public health authorities of a multidimensional response to the emergency.

Before getting back on track and looking at traditional health measures for combating pathogenic illness, let's briefly mention one final instance of community involvement in this book; that of the public's involvement in its writing.

PASCAL AND

LITERARY COMPOSITION

The Provincial Letters

———

In this book, we will focus on Pascal as an example of someone who lived in and thought deeply about a time of transition between paradigms. However, there is one other topic on which his activities can shed light, the art of writing.

In 1656, Pascal was called upon by the religious order with which he was affiliated to write a satire defending it from the abusive treatment it was receiving at the hands of the Jesuits. Under the guise of writing letters from Paris to a country relative, he produced *The Provincial Letters*, which masterfully vindicated his order. In the second transition, we will provide a few more details on the book. Here, though, what I want to highlight is how he wrote this text. A friend of Pascal's described the process of composition. to the French literary critic Boileau. Pascal wanted the letters to be funny, and he consulted friends to make sure his jibes were hitting home.

> When he [Pascal] had written a letter he came and read it to them [his friends, Nicole, Arnauld, Dubois, Saint-Gilles, etc.] and if they found that a single one of the company was unmoved and remained unsmiling when all the others acclaimed it, Pascal rewrote it and kept on revising it until it satisfied everybody.[126]

Another friend noted about the separate letters that Pascal "rewrote several of them as many as seven or eight times in order to bring them to the state of perfection in which we have them."[127]

We see Pascal revised his writing in line with audience response. He sought to move, charm, and educate his readers. There was no way he could judge whether he was reaching his goals by remaining at his desk. He had to read his works aloud, watching the expressions and reactions of his listeners, then consulting with them after he had finished to see whether he was eliciting the effects he sought. When he fell short, he trimmed, expanded or redid each piece until he had a draft that was completely compelling.

Note, too, that he did not only unbosom himself to one intimate, but read versions to a circle of friends, from whom he could get the range of possible reactions he might anticipate from the general reading public.

Something similar is operating here. My cowriter and myself test our thoughts and writings on health in atmospheres in which feedback is essential.

For my part, I run study groups on different health issues. In these settings, each member offers insights from his or her own experience. When I present my thoughts, I do so encouraging constructive criticism, which helps me refine, rethink, and occasionally abandon my positions. As I see it, everyone has something to contribute, even if it is only to point out wrong directions taken which the contributor now regrets. All the major ideas in this book have gone through such a refining fire.

My co-author, Feast, belongs to a group of writers called the Unbearables, who concentrate on performances in which the authors work together toward integrated effects. In their *Unbearable Seance*, for example, held at Shalom's Fusion Arts Club in 1996, the spooky ambiance of a spiritualist session was evoked as one author after another called up the ghost of a deceased literary great. In the weeks leading up to the event, the performing writers read their pieces to their fellows, rebuilding and rethinking their compositions as they hear the comments of peers. Feast, too, has taken some parts of this book to his circle as a way to gauge their value.

Thus, it can be said that collective input, which is so necessary for the successful prosecution of a public health program, also plays a part in the composition of this book.

PART II

TRADITIONAL TREATMENTS

Preliminary Thoughts
on Germ Vectors

Traditional therapies, like better organizations of public health, are the products of collective work. Over the years, groups of scientists have built up a body of knowledge of how germs act and what treatments can interfere with their proliferation. We want to look at this knowledge in this section.

Before getting into specific therapies that have been formulated to handle pathogens, however, it might be worthwhile to say some general things about germs. What we are particularly interested in assaying is the question of why epidemics take place. What sends a germ on a path of destruction?

There are two ways by which a new, virulent pathogen can surface inside the human family. It can arise by mutation or alteration of a microbe that already has been in contact with humans or it can jump from another species into a human population.

To understand how the first situation comes to pass we need to consider how pathogens reproduce. For simplicity's sake, we will confine our discussion to bacteria.

Bacteria do not mate. They produce offspring by dividing. A daughter cell is given a complete match of the mother's chromosomes. Now this type of reproduction could introduce problems in terms of the bacteria's adaptation to the environment. In sexual reproduction, where the new generation is composed of a mix of mother's and father's genes, a variety of offspring with different characteristics are created. This variety makes the species adaptable. If conditions change, certain individuals born may have traits that are particularly congruent with new conditions, and so as the parents of the new generation, they will redirect the species toward now more fitting parameters.

It would seem a bacterium, producing endless clones, lacks this advantage. To get around this limitation, bacteria participate in the exchange and incorporation of genetic material between adult cells. In bacteria,

> genes may be transferred in the form of dissolved DNA molecules or on plasmids (parts of cells). Or one of the two to four identical chromosomes of a bacterium may be transferred via a temporary bridge ("conjugation"), or also by means of a special carrier, in particular, a virus.[1]

This ability to switch genes means that bacteria can quickly adapt themselves to new conditions. If for example, bacteria are in a person being treated with a particular antibiotic, and one group of bacteria has a gene that confers immunity to this drug, then, the group may quickly pass copies of this gene over to their unprotected brothers to help them resist. Bacteria (and viruses) are constantly swapping genes among themselves, not only in respect to crises, as when they are meeting an antibiotic challenge, but as an everyday occurrence. They create new variants that may or may not survive.

Let us suppose a bacterium arises among previously benign microbes, that will kill its human host. Suppose further it lacks an animal reservoir and is spread from person to person. Its chances of long-term survival depend on the nature of the group in which it crops up. If, for instance, this lethal bacterium appears in a band of Neolithic hunters, whose contacts with other bands would be few and far between, it may kill the whole group and then itself disappear since it no longer has a host to transport it.

It has been shown, in fact, that virulent diseases can only exist for a long time in densely populated areas. Calculations of the number of people needed to support a disease have been attempted. It has been estimated, for example, that the less-threatening illness measles needs seven thousand susceptible people available at all times for it to continue in a group. "It turns out that the minimal population needed to keep measles going in a modern city is about half a million."[2]

Of course, there are few or no diseases as lethal as the one we imagined wiping out a hunter band. No disease is 100 percent lethal. (A possible exception may be pneumonic plague.) And no disease will take root in all comers. Sickness, like predators, tends to single out the young, old, and infirm.

So, not only does there have to be a sufficiently large population for a disease to strike, that population have to hold an adequate number of hosts with untried or weakened immunity. This is why epidemics usually occur with exceptional conditions, such a famine, which depresses health levels below normal variations, or a war, which draws the able-bodied out of the population. When pathogens are presented a short-term opportunity, variant strains that can exploit it will always arise or will increase from formerly low numbers."[3] The variant strains, we can suppose, proliferate quickly, not only reproducing like mad, but transferring genes for virulence to related strains, so they too can take advantage of the occasion.

Judging by this information, we might conclude: *The society most resistant to bioterrorism may well be the one in which the citizens have the best record for maintaining superior health,* not the one that possesses the best disease treatment programs!

The second way an epidemic can get started is by transference from another species. We saw how, in an untoward situation where an ecosystem was disrupted, a interspecies-microbe leap took place. As described earlier, when DDT made it possible to eliminate a particular group of weeds in Argentina, in the weeds' place grew a less noxious grass, the favorite meal of a rare field mouse. The mouse increased in numbers and range, intruding into human habitations. The virus, which causes Junín fever, that had been happily and harmlessly residing in this rodent, attempted, much like a pirate boarding a merchantman, to invade the new human host to which it was increasingly exposed. This caused catastrophic effects, *because the virus was not outfitted to live in humans.* Nor is the human immune system prepared to deal with this germ, which previously has not come into contact with.

This final point needs emphasis. As William McNeill has shown in his study of the impact of epidemics, over centuries particular germs find a modus vivendi with humankind. In this balanced state, the germ will not kill the host, a counterproductive move on its part anyway, but merely debilitate him or her to a limited degree, while it lives off what it can scrounge. However, when a disease enters a "virgin" population, one that has never had experience with this microbe and thus been able to establish a working relationship, serious devastation results.

This is what happened in the ancient world when there began to be contacts between what had been isolated civilizations existing in China, India, and Europe. Between AD 165 and AD 180, such a devastating epidemic hit the Roman Empire. McNeill surmises it was an illness previously unknown in the territory.

Despite the scanty evidence it is reasonable to conclude that the disease was new to Mediterranean populations, and behaved as infections are wont to do when they break in upon virgin populations that entirely lack inherited or acquired resistances. Mortality, in other words, was heavy.[4]

So, we have indicated the two natural ways in which deadly germs suddenly become a threat to humans. However, particularly since the twentieth century, humankind has given pathogens a hand by using military means to start epidemics.

It is the role of traditional medicine to find ways to combat outbreaks no matter how they start.

Traditional Means
of Germ Control

Let us not flatter ourselves in the face of our ancestors, believing that before the advent of modern medicine, they were the hapless victims of any diseases that came along, panicking and dying with no recourse except prayer. As we noted, when a new disease breaks in on a "virgin" population, there is a period of shattering death and destruction. After a while, the disease becomes less harrowing as natural immunities develop. A disease like measles, which once cut a swath of death through whole communities, becomes confined to children, who have not had a chance to build tolerance. It is not only immunity, however, which shields an immured people, but their putting into force concrete public health measures.

Take the case, reported by McNeill, of the Manchurian tribesmen, who lived in the vicinity of marmots, a small rodent who sometimes harbored bubonic plague germs. An examination of the "superstitions" that guided the tribesmen in the early twentieth century indicates that, without recognizing marmots' carrier status, they were able to ward off infection. For the Manchurians,

> trapping was taboo; a marmot could only be shot. An animal that moved sluggishly was untouchable, and if a marmot colony showed signs of sickness, custom required the human community to strike its tents and move away to avoid bad luck.[5]

Common sense, public health-supported precautions are still useful in preventing disease spread. Although elsewhere we have registered some reservations about the ideas that AIDS is easily transmitted sexually, there is no question that a switch to safe sex practices on the part of United States homosexuals, influenced by the AIDS scare, made a dent in the spread of STDs. Here the changed folkways of a sexual minority rolled back the spread of syphilis, gonorrhea, and other sexually transmitted illnesses.

The reigning United States medical mindset shortchanges public health and folk measures in favor of drug treatment as the way to go in beating diseases. The healthcare system's tendency to put all its eggs in the drug basket has been decried by a number of physicians groups who argue that, even if vaccines and antibiotics were more reliable than they are, they will not be able to avert biological tragedies that may come about with the appearance of new plagues.

In this section, we will look critically at two weaknesses of modern drug-centered treatments of dire illnesses. We will see that drugs and vaccines now available are not all that safe or reliable (and when given in childhood may decenter the immune system). We will also see that too much reliance on pharmaceutical products is not the savviest way to avert the health disaster new diseases are likely to provoke.

None of which is to say that drugs are to be eschewed altogether or even that those that can have major side effects are never to be taken in emergency situations. Again and again drugs have been life savers. Their value to our health is not in question.

And yet, in the pages that follow we will often have to take the offensive, showing some of the less positive features of pharmaceuticals and traditional medicine, simply because the mainstream media assiduously avoids the down side, leaving the public with an unbalanced understanding. As we will see, the media is not the only institution that has done science a disservice in ill-informed attempts to uphold its virtues.

We will begin by looking at the vaccines used to guard against anthrax, ones that already have had a trial run during the Gulf War. Then we turn to one of the most popular antivirals, ribavirin, and examine its validity in fighting infections. Next we look at vaccines in general, the philosophy behind them, and their effects not only on germs but on the long-term health of the protected human. We then move to a consideration of how vaccines have sometimes been promoted by falsifying the historical record. Moreover, when persuasion doesn't work when used on parents of children who the government wants vaccinated, then the court system gets involved. We end by making a number of moderate recommendations on vaccine use, all stemming from a belief that vaccination should only be used as an occasional supplement to aid naturally boosted immunity.

Anthrax: The Vaccine

S ome have argued that the best way to understand a society is to observe where things don't add up. Those areas indicate strains that will eventually cause innovation or breakdown. In the United States, there is the glaring contradiction between a respected, well-funded scientific establishment and the set of institutions, such as the political structure, that provides science's funding, and then utilize scientific findings with a reckless disregard for the field's procedures, perspective, and ethos.

First, we will see how the shoddy actions of the military in administering the anthrax vaccine seemed to have endangered soldiers' health, then we'll look at the paucity of tests on the vaccine, which cleared it for widespread use. From there, we quickly survey the possibility the vaccine may have illness-provoking additives, that out-of-date vaccines have been administered in the past, and that the vaccine is not relevant to the type of germs that will be employed by terrorists or military enemies. We end by seeing whether the vaccine is implicated in Gulf War illnesses.

What we have in mind in relation to the first point is the situation that came about when United States troops were given anthrax vaccine, preparatory to their going into the field against Iraq. The vaccine had never been employed on such scale, having previously only occasionally been administered to those that worked with animals. Inoculating hundreds of thousands of troops presented an opportunity to test the drug's mettle.

If scientists had been in control, a careful monitoring of the inoculees could have been undertaken and the drug's effects could have been rigorously assessed in hopes of working on its improvement. Instead the military was in charge. The armed forces are set up to win battles, not conduct scientific investigations. Where medical research depends on open, collegial sharing of all information in a democratic atmosphere, the military relies on cover-ups, the seclusion of knowledge from all but the higher-ups, and a hierarchical chain of command.

A study by Garth Nicolson and colleagues from the Institute for Molecular Medicine in Huntington Beach, California, and Parkview Hospital in Brunswick, Maryland, brings out some of the counter-scientific procedures indulged in when the military administered the drugs. Accepted procedure for evaluating vaccines, according to Nicolson et al., is for an independent contractor (independent from the agency providing the dosage) to evaluate the inoculated, recording *any* adverse reactions, which are then tabulated and sent to the FDA's Vaccine Adverse Event Reporting System (VAERS). "In the case of anthrax vaccine, military physicians were instructed that only certain adverse effects could be vaccine reactions…and others such as joint pain, cognitive disturbances, etc. could not be due to the vaccine."[6] The military doctors had no access to data on the varied side effects recorded for the vaccine, including joint pains and others they were told not to report, nor did they look for long-term effects. The upshot was "only reactions that resulted in hospitalization or immediate loss of twenty-four hours of duty time were reported."[7] With adverse symptoms delimited *in advance*, there was little chance for a discovery of the broad range of possible vaccine effects.

Literalist doctors took this so far as to discourage soldiers from reporting illnesses when they didn't fit the bill as laid out in their instructions. The case of Air Force pilot Captain Michelle Piel illustrates this situation. After her first anthrax inoculation, her arm went numb. Some time later, her head filled with fluid. Her condition was so bad she was grounded. Her doctor diagnosed this as a middle ear infection. When she got a second shot, she had the same numbness and symptoms of inner ear infection. Now, she suffered dizzy spells that kept her from driving and reading. The doctors decided to discontinue the anthrax shots. Hearing about the need for VAERS reports in such circumstances, she approached the chief flight surgeon, thinking he might help her fill one out. However, the "surgeon said her particular reaction[s] didn't fall within the criteria of reportable events."[8] She voiced an understandable reaction. "It didn't make sense to me.… I was too sick to fly. I was too sick to get another shot. But my illness wasn't reportable on a VAERS form."[9]

Another feature of textbook-pure science is accurate record-keeping. How did the military do on that score? "In contrast to previous wars, service personnel were not allowed to keep a record of these vaccinations, and according to the DOD [Department of Defense] the shot records of hundreds of thousands of deployed personnel have since disappeared."[10] Health personnel were threatened with court martial if they were found keeping their own records. Thus it would be difficult to know if there was a close connection between getting a shot and the onset of illness.

This was compounded by the fact that vaccines were not given according to Hoyle. We saw already how TB patients can screw up both their own health and that of a susceptible population (since they give birth to extra-resistant germs) by not following their drug regimen rigorously. God help us when such neglectful and aberrant behavior becomes institutionalized.

> After passing their physical exams, they [military personnel preparing to go to the Gulf] received several types of vaccinations, mostly with commercially available vaccines. In the Persian Gulf area this was usually done by administering as many as two dozen vaccine doses over a period of a few days, even if the vaccines were normally required to be given over a course of several months to over a year.[11]

As Nicolson and colleagues make clear, aside from flying in the face of scientific procedure and possibly erasing the positive disease-combating effects the vaccines might have, massive doses of vaccines "can result in immune depression and leave individuals susceptible to opportunistic infections, such as types the vaccine were supposed to protect against."[12]

In light of military physicians' ignorance of the full range of possible adverse side effects to the vaccine, it is not surprising that these doctors often pooh-poohed complaints of vaccinated men. A reporter for the *Cleveland Free Times* describes the case of local man Tom Colosimo, a seven-year Air Force vet, and former body builder, who was given anthrax inoculations from February 1998 to September 1999. (Since the shots were spaced in time and not mixed with other inoculations, it has been easier to gauge their effects than it is to study the effects of those given in a jumbled sequence.) The first shot made him feel dizzy and fatigued. After the second shot, he broke out with cysts on his face and head. "A doctor told him the cysts might be caused by sweat because Colosimo was working out so much."[13] After taking his fourth shot, he was sent to Kuwait, where he felt nausea and chest pains. "In eight weeks, he shed forty pounds."[14]

Back home, his physical deterioration became worse, with frequent blackouts and dizziness, leading to periods of hospitalization. Given that these symptoms weren't recognized as related to his vaccinations—remember Airwoman Piel also suffered dizziness, which her doctor said couldn't be ascribed to the vaccine—he "developed a reputation as a malingerer."[15] Once when the police came to the base, responding to a call that Colosimo had collapsed, the police sergeant "said he was sick of playing games…and accused him of faking his illness."[16]

Colosimo was eventually vindicated when the military admitted it was wrong about him. Marine Major General Randall West, in testimony before a House Subcommittee, stated, "Unfortunately the doctors do believe that…Colosimo's problems were caused by the anthrax vaccine."[17] (2) Yet, General West qualified his admission in this way, "Of all the people that were here today [various military personnel claiming to have suffered adverse effects from the vaccination] there was only one person who had a medical diagnosis that directly links it to the anthrax vaccine."[18] This one person was Colosimo.

The general is claiming that ill effects from the vaccine are nearly unheard of occurrences. This itself is not in dispute here. Rather we are saying that *this or any other general statement about the effect of the vaccine on Gulf War participants is valueless* given the complete failure of the military medical system to follow accepted scientific procedures in administering and keeping track of the results of the vaccine.

Thinking further, it may be said that this situation is highly ironic, in that the military establishment that here shows itself so impervious to the standards of sound medical practice was once at the cutting edge of health care. As McNeill documents, in the 1700s when various scientists argued that improvements in sanitation would stop the spread of illness, armies and navies were the places where experiments in cleanliness were pioneered. "European armies, being the pets and playthings of Europe's crowned heads, were both too valuable in the eyes of authority and too amenable to control from above not to benefit from a growing corpus of sanitary regulations."[19] Long before cities and towns received clean drinking water, adequate sewage disposal, and pure food, these were granted to troops, whose health improvements gave evidence of the utility of such adjustments.

Now, however, the military seems to have grown woefully lax in attending to medical matters. And when individuals call attention to problems and indiscrepancies, and where in a scientific atmosphere their grievances would be dispassionately assessed, in the prevailing military climate these complainants bear a punitive brunt. We saw that in how, at first, Colosimo was branded a malingerer. Two more recent cases show the same intolerance on the part of defense authorities who refuse to entertain any objections to orders.

In October 2000, Captain John Buck, a military doctor stationed at Kessler Air Force base in Mississippi, refused to take anthrax inoculations. He gave his reasons, "I view this as an investigational vaccine being used in an off-label fashion."[20] That is, to his mind, there was wholesale administration of a vaccine that had never been adequately tested. Buck argued further, that if, as an officer, he understood the necessity of following orders, as a doctor, he appreciated the importance of respecting patients' rights and testing drugs on a small sample before exposing a large population to it. Buck was facing court martial for his stance. Whatever his fate as of January 2002, *102 military personnel had already been court-martialed* for refusing vaccination.

Earlier in the year, Air Force Major Sonnie Bates from Dover Air Force base in Delaware took the same position by refusing anthrax vaccine. His unwillingness to get vaccinated was not based in medical scruple, but more pragmatic concerns. "Medical records obtained by CBS News [which was doing a piece on Bates's case] show that more than one hundred service members [at his base] reported the vaccine made them ill. Some pilots became so sick they were grounded."[21] As in the Colosimo incident, charges flew that those who became sick were simply trying to escape duty. Moreover, Bates reports that other personnel came to him, saying, "Major, the doctor told me if I talk about anthrax that I'll be facing medical discharge."[22]

Bates grounded his worries in what he understood about military boondoggles. He knew the one plant making the vaccine had been repeatedly cited for safety violations, and, as he put it, "There is a difference between being willing to give your life and sacrificing your health over a mismanaged government contract."[23]

The plant Bates was alarmed about is owned by BioPort, which is located in Lansing, Michigan. The facility had been in the possession of the state, but was so plagued with safety problems that the government unloaded it in 1997. The group that bought the factory was headed by Fuad El-Hibri, a German-born businessman of Lebanese extraction who is now a

United States citizen. Some improprieties were suspected in that two weeks after BioPort took over the biological establishment, the firm signed a contract with the Pentagon for $45 million to supply anthrax vaccine (called AVA). The suspicions about the firm were based on the fact that retired Admiral William Crowe, Jr., who had been head of the Joint Chiefs of Staff as well as Ambassador to Britain—El-Hibri had owned a British biological corporation—"was given 12 percent to 13 percent of the company in exchange for a 'token amount' and BioPort's use of his name."[24]

It has been reported that Admiral Crowe had been lobbying the DoD in El-Hibri's behalf from the beginning.

As with so many Pentagon contracts, there were cost overruns. In 1999, the government granted BioPort an additional $24.1 million for the original contract and upped the payment for individual doses from 200 percent to 500 percent for fewer doses.[25]

Although these seemingly shady goings-on give one pause, they are not germane to the major question being raised here: Is the anthrax vaccine safe? We should begin by being clear that, as the CDC notices, the few studies that have been done, give AVA a clean bill of health. One report looked at the reactions of inoculees to the vaccine during the Korean War. "Most reported [adverse health] events were localized, minor and self limited," with only 0.3 percent experiencing a full day's loss from duty.[26] As to long-term ill effects, which the Korean War study did not look into, an examination of workers at the United States biowarfare base at Fort Detrick (who have to be inoculated for germs they are working with) found there were no unusual illnesses or conditions associated with AVA over a long time span. Lastly, two studies of Gulf War veterans who had been given the vaccine showed "no association" between taking the anthrax vaccination and Gulf War syndrome.[27]

These studies have been positive, although one can't help remarking on the paucity of examinations of a vaccine that is being distributed so widely in the armed forces. As Captain Buck noted, it seems unwise to use a drug so widely on which only a few studies have been done. Moreover, a different examination of the effect of the vaccine on the Gulf War military, cited in the Cleveland paper, looked at Kansas City veterans and "found that 34 percent of those who were vaccinated and deployed met the definition for Gulf War syndrome, compared to 4 percent of Gulf War–era veterans who were not deployed and did not receive the vaccine."[28] On top of that, 12 percent of veterans who were not sent to the theater of war but who *did* receive the vaccine came down with the Gulf War medical condition. This, let us note, is far from solid proof that the syndrome is tied to the vaccination, in that there are many other factors that may play a part in generation of the disease condition. We can say, however, that evidence on the implication of the anthrax vaccine in short- and long-term illness is inconclusive at best.

You might note, by the way, that the vaccine was approved in 1970 before tests to meet FDA approval were required. "In the case of the anthrax vaccine, long-term safety date were not supplied with the license application, and none has as yet been supplied to the FDA."[29]

Vaccines are often produced with weakened or dead germs of the disease to be guarded against. AVA itself doesn't use whole anthrax bacteria but cellular bits from the *B. anthracis* that are found in edemal (intercellular) fluid of infected animals. This doesn't mean that these bits are directly injected into the blood, because the germ—and this is the case with all vaccines—has to be carried by different agents in the vaccine, called "adjuvants." In AVA, the major adjuvants is aluminum hydroxide.

There are some researchers who feel agents such as aluminum hydroxide may themselves cause a problem.[30] Nonetheless, an outcry around the preparation used to safeguard Gulf War troops turns not on the adjuvant that have been authorized but on the possibility that unapproved ones were added. In fact, an investigation by Congressman Jack Metcalf (assisted by the federal government's General Accounting Office or GAO), revealed in a hearing held in November 2001 that squalene, an oil used in the processing of cholesterol, was found in tested anthrax vaccine. It was suggested that this oil might have also appeared in the vaccine given to those going into battle in the Gulf War. What is at issue is not that squalene causes some particular problem, but that as an untested additive, no one knows what squalene's effect might be.

Metcalf's investigation took three years, partly because of the obstructive attitude of the Defense Department. "GAO also found Peter Collis, DOD official who headed vaccine efforts, refused to cooperate with them."[31] Overall, the GAO found "a pattern of deception," with the Pentagon changing its story whenever it was faced with evidence that former stories didn't hold water.

Not only has military authority been charged with trying out experimental versions of the vaccine, ones laced with an untried adjuvant, but it has been further accused of being in such a hurry to get its forces inoculated that it used outdated medicines. Given the outcry around the use of the vaccine, in 1998 some of the remaining lots from AVA used to inoculate the troops were tested. Only six out of thirty-one lots retested were potent. Partially this was because the vaccine had expired. However, it was still being treated by the military as if were ready for use, and the lots had been redated once it had expired, not only once but sometimes twice, after a second expiration. "The question was raised whether expired or failed vaccine lots were used for vaccinating military personnel during the Gulf War."[32] If, as it seemed to be, standard procedure was to keep redating vaccines (perhaps so they wouldn't go to waste), then it is not unlikely—and this is what the researchers retesting the vaccine concluded—that out-of-date and hence ineffective vaccines were given to the fighting troops.

Aside from these possible problems with the vaccine, there is the further question of whether, even in its approved state, it would be effective against the type of anthrax a germ warfare-toting opponent is likely to throw at our military. As already noted, the most effective route for spreading anthrax is via airborne spores. Soldiers breathing in the bacteria would contract inhalational anthrax, the deadliest form of the infection. This is the type of infection that recently killed a reporter, two postal employees, and a New York hospital worker. However, the vaccine has not proven itself against this form of the disease. "A study of an earlier anthrax vaccine…found that it protected humans against anthrax absorbed through the skin, but could not determine its efficacy against inhaled anthrax."[33]

Let's say, for the time being, that AVA could cope with inhalational anthrax. Even then, the vaccine would only be useful against straw enemies who had nothing in their arsenal except the simple airborne spores. As the group Doctors for Disaster Preparedness point out, "An additional threat in the context of biological warfare is the potential use of genetically engineered strains, against which both vaccine and antibiotics may be ineffective."[34] We now know that both Soviet biowarfare and Iraqi laboratories developed new, more potent strains of anthrax. Further, it seems only the most unsophisticated enemy would rely on one germ for its attack. The weapon of choice now is the so-called "Russian Doll Cocktail." This is "an aerosolized BW and chemical mixture that is designed to inhibit and overwhelm the body's defensive abilities."[35] Not only would such a cocktail contain more than one disease agent, but it would enclose a number of drugs that weaken immunity, allowing the diseases a freer hand. Nicolson and colleagues comment,

> The United States military's strategy of defense against BW agents is prior immunization using multiple vaccines. Unfortunately, this can only be successful if the exact BW agents likely to be encountered are known in great detail and for some time in advance of exposure.[36]

Such forewarning is hard to come by, but without it, these experts argue, there is little chance immunization will offer much protection.

Let us end this section by returning to the question of the Gulf War syndrome (also known as Gulf War Illnesses to indicate their may be more than one disease involved here). This condition is characterized by chronic fatigue, headaches, nausea, cognitive and gastrointestinal dysfunctions, fever, joint aches, muscle pains and other symptoms. The jury is still out on what is behind this medical condition, and the correlative study we noted, which sought to link anthrax inoculations to the syndrome, was not convincing. However, we should think about what we mentioned earlier about the way multiple immunizations weaken the immune system, and some say this is behind the syndrome. This point would not make AVA alone responsible for the illness, but rather a contributor that works in conjunction with all the other vaccines passed out. If we tie this to reports on the anthrax vaccine by British Gulf War veterans, the only group that did test the vaccines used on the troops, which found the vaccine was contaminated with unknown microorganisms, we might agree with Dr. Nicolson and his colleagues, who suspect that the anthrax vaccine (along with others given in such haste) had *a part* to play in causing the syndrome. Note well, the Nicolson study does not lay the whole illness at the door of AVA or any of the other administered vaccines, but simply sees it and them as vital contributing factors. The scientists summarize their opinion in this way:

> If stress is added to multiple vaccines given at once, plus chemical and other toxic exposures encountered during the Gulf War, then immune suppression and opportunistic infections could be likely outcome in at least a subset of the military personnel that subsequently came down with GWI [Gulf War Illnesses].[37]

At the moment, these problems with AVA are of most concern to military personnel since they are ones who, even today, face vaccinations as preparation for going into battle against bioweapon-armed foes. The general population, which is susceptible to random terrorist attacks with aerosolized anthrax, as the five deaths in 2001 showed, will be more affected by the antibiotics that are available to head off anthrax once a person has been infected with it. So let us look at those now.

Anthrax:
The Antibiotic Ciprofloxacin

The October 2001 infection of a number of Americans by anthrax spores, which they were exposed to through the mail and which made them either deathly ill or killed them outright, caused a panic in both the public and public health agencies. Although the threat was diabolically real, many people went overboard by dosing themselves with the antibiotic ciprofloxacin when there was no chance they had been exposed to the disease. Moreover, the government was recommending people take this potent drug when, as it turned out, they would have been much better off taking equally effective, less powerful concoctions, such as penicillin.

Given the unprecedented circumstances, the shock and overreaction were certainly understandable, perhaps, unavoidable; but before we are faced with another such incident, we need to be clearer about the treatment possibilities.

Recall for a moment what people thought and the news reported when the first anthrax-laden letters were discovered. It seemed to be the obvious work of al-Qaida, the terrorist network that destroyed the World Trade Centers. Such thinking might be called an adoption of a worst case scenario. If this attribution were accurate, it would indicate Osama bin Laden's group was even more insidious than it had so far shown itself to be and was supplied with not only military but biological weapons. A frightening thought. As it turns out, though, the fact that the form of anthrax used, called the Ames strain, had been created in United States laboratories, along with other evidence, indicates the mailing was done by a disgruntled American scientist, who was using the recent Arab terrorism as a cover for his own nefarious deeds. In fact, the British newspaper, *The Guardian*, reported at the end of July 2002, that Dr. Barbara Rosenberg, biowarfare expert employed by the Federation of American Scientists, "claimed that biodefense experts had told the FBI the identity of a likely suspect but that the bureau was keeping it secret, possibly because the suspect knows too much about United States experimentation with germ warfare."[38]

The same type of worst-case scenario was imagined in terms of the dangers stemming from the anthrax attacks. The CDC and other agencies were prescribing ciprofloxacin. In a directive to public health agencies, for example, the CDC said, "You have been given this drug [ciprofloxacin] for protection against possible exposure to an infection-causing bacteria.... Take this medicine as prescribed, one tablet by mouth, two times a day."[39]

Yet, as an article in the *Washington Post* points out, ciprofloxacin (known as Cipro) was never meant to be an all-purpose antibiotic against anthrax. *Bacillus anthracis* is amenable to treatment with several other antibiotic drugs, including penicillin, amoxicillin, doxycycline, tetracycline, clarithromycin, and clindamycin. Cipro was created out of fear that terrorists would strike with a form of anthrax that was bioengineered to resist the usual antibiotics. Fear of the use of an extra-deadly anthrax was so great that the government rushed the new drug through the FDA's approval process, relying on a single animal study to vouch for its effectiveness. Moreover, there wasn't time to ascertain exactly how long the drug needed to be administered to the exposed. When the booby-trapped letters began appearing, government medical agencies assumed their apprehensions were being realized, a antibiotic-resistant anthrax was in play. They prescribed Cipro as drug of choice. The *Post* writer, Shankar Vedantam, explains that it turned out

> the attack involved a strain of anthrax that was not bioengineered to be impervious to the other drugs [such as penicillin], which are safer and cheaper. And the number of people exposed and sickened was far fewer than planners had feared.... The disparity between the imagined attack and the real one underscores the difficulty of formulating public health measures against little-known bioweapons, and the very real danger that some cures can cause more harm than the bioweapons themselves.[40]

We need to unpack this last clause. There are four possible harms that came from the decision to prescribe Cipro for those who thought they were exposed to inhalational anthrax: (1) people were self medicating with the drug when they hadn't been exposed to the bacteria, (2) Cipro is more potent than the other antibiotics used against anthrax and consequently can produce more devastating side effects, (3) a widespread use of the drug—and, note, Cipro is a standard treatment for other diseases, such as TB, when all else fails—will encourage the growth of resistant strains of bacteria, and (4) since Cipro had not been fully studied, it is not known how long a course of treatment with it should run, but the government advocated sixty days of pill-taking, beyond what many feel is safe.

SELF-MEDICATION

After the postal attacks, "when the public discovered that Cipro was the only approved medication for inhalational anthrax, demand soared."[41] Not only did people beg their doctors for prescriptions, but they began buying it over the Internet and dosing themselves. The CDC reports that about 32,000 people have started taking antibiotics to prevent anthrax since October 8, 2001, and about 5,000 have been instructed to take a sixty-day course.[42]

One catalyst provoking people that were feeling sick to reach for the Cipro was the resemblance between the symptoms at the onset of influenza and anthrax. "The first signs of inhaled anthrax are cough, headache, fever, and a general sense of feeling lousy. However, these are precisely the same symptoms of flu and a long list of viruses that cause respiratory infections."[43]

What is nerve-wracking is that effective treatment against inhalational anthrax has to be started soon after exposure. But, to distinguish the deadly disease from garden-variety flu a blood test is needed, and this takes a few days to process. Aside from that, an infected person's blood test may be misleading because the anthrax bacteria doesn't always proliferate in the first days after contraction of the germ. Thus, well-meaning doctors may have misdiagnosed flu as anthrax, prescribing accordingly, given the danger they might be putting their patients in if they failed to recognize the bacteria.

SIDE EFFECTS

As a rule of thumb, we can say the stronger a medication proves itself against microbes, the more toxic it is to the human body. (Don't get me wrong. Of course, there are circumstances when the taking of such powerful medications is to be recommended.) Since Cipro is a super-charged antibiotic, it stands to reason it may have harsh side effects. The most common adverse reactions to Cipro are a mild upset stomach, diarrhea, vomiting, and headache. Rarer problems are difficulty in breathing, skin rashes, blood in urine, and, more damaging, seizures, vision changes, and pain or rupture of tendons.

It's worth noting that a recent article in *Annals of Pharmacotherapy* zeroed in on how harmful the side effects of Cipro and related drugs from the fluroquinolone family can be. (This family does not include penicillin and others we mentioned as safer antibiotics to which anthrax responds.) This was not an examination of anyone taking the drugs but only of those who suffered adverse effects, such as tingling, numbness, and burning pain or spasms, all symptoms connected to dysfunctions in the peripheral nervous system.

The study, done by Jay S. Cohen, MD, a professor at the University of California, San Diego, surveyed forty-five patients with these effects and found 93 percent of sufferers had these peripheral symptoms compounded by ones that stemmed from disturbance of other major bodily systems, such as tendon rupture (relating to the musco-skeletal system) or impaired cognitive functions (relating to the central nervous system). The bulk of the cases were severe (80 percent), and a majority (58 percent) had symptoms that lasted longer than a year. Cohen mentions further, a point that will sound familiar after our study of reactions in the military, that "eighteen patients stated that their physicians either failed to recognize or dismissed the significance of their neuropathies.… At least four patients were told to continue taking the antibiotics despite complaining of adverse events."[44]

Looking over patients' reactions to the recent surge in Cipro taking that occurred in connection with the postal attacks, the CDC's *Morbidity and Mortality Weekly Report*, stated that about one in five people taking ciprofloxacin or doxycycline (another fluroquinolone medication) against anthrax reports side effects such as itching, breathing problems or swelling of face, neck, or throat. In line with these figures, 95 (19 percent) of the 490 respondents to a questionnaire reported one or more adverse effect. About 2 percent reported symptoms that indicated a severe allergic reaction. Nancy Rosenstein, MD, from the CDC, was asked whether such a high amount of adverse reactions, nearly a fifth of those treated, was to be expected. She said, "While the number may be slightly higher than what's in the *PDR* [*Physician's Desk Reference*], it is still within the realm of the same as other reports."[45]

With such hazards associated with the antibiotic, one has to be careful in taking it, not doing so unless there is a good chance one has come in contact with the disease and that the anthrax is a antibiotic-resistant form. Moreover, once one is taking Cipro, one has to monitor closely what other drugs or foods are being consumed. The CDC notes that anyone taking Cipro should not take any antacids, vitamins, iron supplements, zinc supplements, sucralfate, blood thinners, theophylline, asthma, or gout medication. Also to be avoided are such foods and beverages as coffee, tea, caffinated soft drinks, and foods containing large amounts of calcium, such as milk, yogurt, or cheese.[46]

Moreover, in most countries Cipro is not licensed for use in pregnancy or for children, where it may cause damage to the cartilage in weight-bearing joints, as experimentally observed in young dogs. *JAMA* notes, "Ciprofloxacin and other fluroquinolones should not be used in children younger than sixteen to eighteen."[47] They make the same recommendation for pregnant women, although the medical association tempers both these statements with the proviso that if either group has been directly exposed to an attack with bio-engineered anthrax, it may be necessary to balance survival against the probability of grim side effects and recommend the antibiotic.

DANGER OF CREATING CIPRO-RESISTANT BACTERIAL STRAINS

As will be recalled, Cipro is a drug of last resort for anthrax, meant to be prescribed against strains of the disease that are resistant to other antibiotics. We've already discussed how germs gain the ability to withstand medications that once would have eliminated them, but let's briefly review that material as a way of leading up to this troubling question: What do we do against bacteria who have become immune to an antibiotic specifically engineered to fight them?

We mentioned the case of a resistant strain of TB that was fostered when patients stopped taking their medications prematurely. A fact sheet from a New Mexico health agency describes what can happen in such a situation, specifically in relation to Cipro. "If the drug doesn't kill all the germs, they might change (mutate) so that they can survive even when you are taking medications. When this happens, the drug will stop working."[48] Only the hardiest bacteria will have survived the assault from Cipro thus far, and, with the discontinuation of the dosage, these will be the template on which the next generation of microbes will model themselves.

Germs are wily when it comes to mutating and gene-exchanging their way out of endangering environments. The parasite that causes malaria, for example, has found a way to escape the ravages of quinine drugs. One of this protozoa's favorite foods is human blood, specifically, hemoglobin (the part of the blood cell that carries oxygen). However, hemoglobin contains iron, which is toxic to the parasite. In the malarial parasite, there are special cavities called vacuoles, in which the iron is sequestered so that it can do no harm to the pathogen. The mode of action of quinine is to inhibit the enzyme that is needed to form vacuoles. "When the drugs are present, the iron is free to diffuse through the rest of the parasite cell, killing it.[49]

However, with the overuse or misuse of quinine-based drugs, new strains of malaria have grown that are unfazed by the medications. A team of researchers at the Picower Institute for Medical Research led by Andrew Slater discovered that these DR parasites "have somehow acquired the ability to avoid concentrating the drugs in their food vacuoles in the first place."[50] That is, just as this germ learned how to compartmentalize iron so it won't interfere with its life, it has found out how to sequester quinine for the same purpose.

We may add, in passing, that a number of bacteria have developed an ingenious method for escaping antibiotics by developing cellular "pumps." A potentially harmful drug is identified as it penetrates the bacterium's cell wall and is efficiently pumped back out before it can do any damage.

Cipro's mode of action is to stop a bacterium from reproducing. According to the drug's manufacturer, Bayer Corporation, "The bactericidal action of ciprofloxacin results from interference with the enzyme DNA gyrase which is needed for the synthesis of bacterial DNA."[51] We can imagine, then, that a mutant form of anthrax could find a way to compartmentalize or pump out Cipro before it took effect. Or perhaps, like influenza, which systematically alters its antigens to avoid detection by antibodies, the anthrax bacteria would find a substitute enzyme with which it could carry on DNA manufacture unaffected by Cipro. In any case, if conditions allow anthrax to evolve, no doubt it will become drug resistant.

On this note, we might add that it is not only by way of the development of MDR anthrax strains that Cipro's ability to heal may be weakened. After all, even factoring in terrorist incidents, anthrax is bound to be a rare disease. Cipro is a multi-purpose drug that has been found to be effective and is already being used successfully against many microorganisms. The FDA has approved its use against such diseases as acute sinusitis (including pneumonial ones), various lower respiratory tract infections, urinary tract infections (including those caused by E. coli), cystitis, intra-abdominal infections, skin infections, bone and joint infections, gonorrhea, typhoid fever, and infectious diarrhea. So, it may be that in treating these other infections Cipro-immune microorganisms will develop.

Wills says, "There is no doubt that effective defenses against even drug-resistant pathogens can continue to be generated, since our knowledge of these pathogens will continue to grow. But as these drugs become more sophisticated, they are also becoming progressively more expensive."[52] Moreover, nowadays there is less lapsed time between development of a new antibiotic and the formation of drug-resistant breeds of bacteria. Thus, while we can keep throwing new drugs at MDR bacteria, it would obviously be better if a tight control on the dispensing of antibiotics and careful monitoring of those taking them made it impossible for superpotent strains to develop in the first place.

LENGTH OF TREATMENT

If patients, such as the alcoholics who stopped taking their TB meds because they interfered with their drinking, welch on their understanding with their doctors by not following through on treatment, it is as if they were breaking an implicit contract. The patient agrees to abide by the doctor's recommendations in exchange for getting the best possible health advice.

The second part of such an agreement turns on the physician's dispensing of sensible counsel. With antibiotics, proper advice would include a judicious assessment of length of treatment. It is necessary that the regimen be continued long enough for a thorough flushing out of disease germs; but at the same time, knowing that all antibiotics can have unwanted side effects, and especially that many, like Cipro, are cumulative (that is, the more you take, the more you risk a negative counterreaction), the course of antibiotics should be no longer than absolutely necessary.

Remember, too, in a point that has been repeatedly brought up in medical literature, that antibiotics not only kill off bad bacteria, such as anthrax, but mow down good bacteria, like those found in the gut, that aid in food digestion. The longer one swallows any antibiotic, the more disturbance there is to beneficial microflora.

So, in prescribing proper dosage during the anthrax panic, the government may have erred on the side of caution. When the FDA considered the best use of Cipro should a terrorist attack occur, the agency's personnel had in the front of their minds the worst case. They were basing their evaluations on a paper published in *JAMA*, which projected deaths from an anthrax blitz on a major city in the range of 130,000 to 3 million unless the exposed received immediate treatment.

And it was not only the size of the devastation that had to be projected, but the length of time those affected would need to take the drug. "No studies had demonstrated that [the decided upon Cipro dosage schedule] was necessary for the kind of attack that actually occurred."[53] Such studies would be difficult to undertake since the time aerosolized anthrax took to produce disease was also unknown. Janet Woodcock, director of the FDA's Center for Drug Evaluation and Research, stated to a *Washington Post* reporter, "The question was, if you've inhaled spores, how long will it be before you can be safely off antibiotics?... People could develop cases weeks away from their exposure."[54]

Crucially, even if what Woodcock admits is a "worst-case scenario" had come true and there had been massive exposure, there was substantial risk to the public in prescribing such a long stint on Cipro, something that had never been previously envisioned. Philip Hanna, anthrax expert from the University of Michigan at Ann Arbor, pointed out that previous studies on Cipro's side effects had never involved taking the drug for more than ten days. "When you start giving it for two months," Hanna said, "that's a whole level of usage that hasn't been proven to be safe."[55] Leigh Thompson, a South Carolina MD, who has had experience with Cipro, went even further in warning against this dosage. Asked about putting people on the sixty-day regimen, he exclaimed, "God, that would be insane."[56]

Again let us try to avoid giving a false impression. The point is not that the FDA's recommendation on dosage is wrong, especially in relation to worse attacks that may lurk over the horizon. If things were going to get as bad as imagined, the sixty-day dosage routine would have been a good stab at a rational response, unavoidable, given the lack of time to develop alternatives.

But that's all supposing the worst case had come to pass. Since it didn't, one wishes that at the onset of the postal assaults the government had waited to get a better feel for the situation before pushing for the most drastic measures. Even though, after the first excitement, the FDA allowed that penicillin and other more moderate drugs might be taken instead of Cipro, it was the first alarm when people were most open to any suggestion to alleviate their panic when ciprofloxacin was set out as a wonder drug. Everyone began clamoring for it. It would seem that the FDA, though well aware of terrorism's dangers, is unmindful of the fact that antibiotics and antivirals have drawbacks, and this is true not only of Cipro, but of the even more commonly prescribed ribavirin, which is next on our agenda.

Ribavirin

Repeatedly, we have come across the name ribavirin in our survey of preventive measures against viral infections. We have seen that it is one of the few treatments suggested for Lassa fever, Argentine hemorrhagic fever, Crimean-Congo fever, and Nipah virus. The Internet health site *Medscape* notes, "Ribavirin has a spectrum of antiviral activity that is broader than that of other currently available antiviral agents."[57] It has proven itself against multiple DNA and RNA viruses. Aside from being useful against the exotic viruses we mentioned, ribavirin is employed against lower respiratory tract infections, such as bronchitis and pneumonia, influenza, genital herpes, hepatitis, and measles, among other illnesses. It can be taken orally, though for bronchial and respiratory infections, the drug is usually given as a mist inhalant. In the latter case, "the medication is put in a special machine to make mist which is then inhaled through an oxygen hood, face mask or oxygen tent. This makes sure the drug reaches deep into the lungs."[58]

Since it is extensively prescribed, a good deal of data has been gathered about ribavirin's side effects, more than we have on Cipro or other drugs that have not gotten wide play. However, in view of the fact that this antiviral is taken by people suffering serious health problems, when deteriorating conditions are witnessed in these patients, it is not easy to distinguish between an adverse reaction to the drug and simply a worsening of the illness. For instance, in connection to patients with severe respiratory tract infections, "death has occurred in twenty patients during or shortly after discontinuance of ribavirin inhalation therapy, but a causal relationship to the drug was not clearly established."[59]

We do know that ribavirin is very commonly associated with an aggravation of respiratory conditions. When given in oral form in connection with interferon alfa-2b (this latter drug is milder in effect),

> about 19 percent of treatment-naive [those who have never taken the drugs before] and 6 percent of treatment-experienced patients receiving combination therapy in clinical studies discontinued therapy because of adverse [especially respiratory] effects."[60]

In particular, when the medicine is being used on asthma or chronic obstructive pulmonary disease, there have been incidents of pulmonary worsening, pain in the chest, and labored breathing. In some cases, decline has led to the patient having to be put on a respirator with the failure of adequate unassisted breathing. When the patient is so far gone in a disease state that he or she is already on a mechanical respirator, inhalation therapy has occasionally interfered with the artificial lungs. Several infants on respirators died when given ribavirin mist. "In these cases, death was attributed to mechanical ventilator malfunction caused by precipitation of the drug within the ventilator apparatus that led to...diminished oxygenation."[61] More simply put, the ribavirin spray leaked into the respirator, blocking enough of the oxygen flow that the child asphyxiated.

Aside from respiratory impairment, the other major problems linked with ribavirin treatment have been cardiovascular. Of note, patients have suffered heart attacks, abnormally low blood pressure, slowed heartbeat, and excessively speeded-up heartbeat. Separate animal experiments have shown cardiac lesions in mice and rats who took the drug for a month, and on rats and monkeys who took it for more extended periods, going up to a half year.

Another occasional side effect is anemia caused by blood poisoning and interference with hemoglobin. On patients suffering this ill effect, "anemia usually was mild and reversible within 2–4 weeks after discontinuance of the drug, although severe anemia, which may require transfusion can occur."[62] Ribavirin accumulates in red blood cells, shortening their lives, and, in some cases, leading to a low count as there is a lag in providing their replacements.

The drug has also been associated with rash, conjunctivitis, and other eye problems as well as with nervous system effects. Three clinical studies found insomnia, depression, and irritability occurring in ranges of 26 percent to 39 percent, 23 percent to 32 percent, and 23 percent to 25 percent of patients who were taking the ribavirin along with interferon alfa-2b.[63] Although long-term effects have not been much studied, animal experiments find the drug can be cancer promoting.

We have been highlighting the more drastic, rarer effects. The more typical and less health-threatening negative effects are an unusual tiredness and fatigue, headaches, loss of appetite, and nausea.

We should also note that this is one drug whose side effects have also been of concern to health personnel, who may breathe in the mist they are administering to their patients, as well as to people visiting the sufferer during therapy. "Some experts and clinicians state that such exposure of pregnant women and possibly those who may become pregnant may represent a risk to the foetus." Although the exact health risks have not been assessed, it has been shown that health care workers do receive a measurable dose of ribavirin while conducting the treatment. It has also come out that "ribavirin can precipitate on contact lenses of health-care personnel exposed to the aerosolized drug, and such precipitation may be associated with conjunctivitis."[65] The Canadian Medical Association notes that fear has been building among nurses and other hospital employees about exposure to ribavirin.

> The anxiety about the risk of exposure has reached such heights that one major pediatric centre does not permit aerosol administration via hood or tent, and another requires extraordinary precautions, including protective clothing, gloves, goggles, and respirators for personnel, and a special containment unit enclosing the infant so that the exhaust air can be filtered.[66]

A biohazard alert that is intended for hospital workers and that originates from the California Department of Health Services echoes the "extraordinary precautions" mentioned above, and goes on to thoroughly describe the isolation and other methods that must be used to keep ribavirin away from any but those needing it. For instance, the alert recommends, "All housekeeping staff should wear protective equipment.... All equipment should be thoroughly cleaned with soap and water.... Linens should be handled with a minimum of shaking, to reduce the release of ribavirin in the room."[67]

Clearly, if healthcare personnel are being told to proceed so cautiously around the medication, it is one that is far from safe. To repeat a former thought, this does not mean we are against this drug. Taking it can be an acceptable risk when one has been beset by one of the hemorrhagic fevers or other deadly viral infections which ribavirin can deter.

Antivirals and
Antibiotics Versus Vaccines

In fact, let us take our last thought a little further to help us compare antibiotics and antivirals, on the one side, and vaccines, on the other.

Once an attendee at one of my seminars asked an important, if slightly naive question. He said something like this, "Gary," he said, "you've been talking about the side effects of this antibiotic. Why don't the damn scientists just make drugs that aren't laced with side effects?"

Think about it this way. Viruses and bacteria have similar structures and overlapping (even identical) parts with human cells. If this weren't true, the germs wouldn't have much of a chance to penetrate our cells and use their machinery (as do viruses) or live off the nutrients that take from our blood and other internal substances (as do bacteria). But this means, because of this similarity, any drug that disrupts viral or bacterial function is more or less certain to interfere with normal cell activity.

Take AZT or any of the chemotherapy drugs, all of which have the same mode of operation, AZT simply being the one with the most killing power of the lot. Each chemotherapeutic agent destroys all growing cells in the body. That means that ideally the agent will kill any new cancer cell or HIV retrovirus (given mainstream doctors' opinion that a retrovirus is behind AIDS.) It also means, and physicians accept this, that it will kill any newly born cell needed for our body's operation, and, specifically, it will kill all the new immune cells, which are the ones generated the fastest. In anti-cancer therapy, at least, this is a gamble that may pay off. If the use of the drugs isn't too protracted, the result may be that the cancer is terminated while the temporary elimination of new immune cells has not been so devastating as to wreck the body beyond repair.

The greater point here is that such drugs offer a tradeoff, which both physicians and informed patients accept. The drug will eliminate the pathogenic agent, but it will also very probably damage the patient's body to a certain, probably manageable extent. Before undergoing treatment, the patient has to decide whether the benefits of the first result sufficiently overbalance the risks of the the second. The whole arrangement is clear-cut and straightforward.

If we look at vaccines, however, we will see that the problems run a little deeper. Here the question is whether the generally used method of immunization, where a weak or dead germ is injected so as to stimulate the production of antibodies that will be able to later cope with the an intruding healthy germ of the same type, is workable at all. On the surface it seems eminently sensible. And even though the basics of immunization were worked out before scientists' knowledge of antibodies and the immune system was very comprehensive, mainstream science still finds vaccine theory in agreement with current notions of biology.

And yet, how does one respond to cases such as this. In the 1950s, polio vaccinations were given to as many children as possible. Yet small polio epidemics continued to occasionally occur. The House Committee on Interstate and Foreign Commerce looked into one such outbreak that was found in Massachusetts in 1961. It was discovered, "There were more paralytic cases in the triple vaccinates than in the unvaccinated."[68]

This may be an anomaly or a case of tainted vaccine. It may also be that so many children were vaccinated that any cases that did occur most likely would occur to those who were immunized. However the possibility we want to explore in the next section is whether such unsettling statistics are symbolic of an overall inadequacy in the theory and practice of vaccines.

Vaccines

"If vaccines stimulate the production of antibodies, and antibodies fight disease," you might ask, "how could vaccination be in error?"

Our reply, which will be given in full at the end of this section, will begin with a discussion of the holistic operation of the immune system. When a disease, one which the immune system eventually routs, enters the body naturally, the production of antibodies is only one part of a multileveled response, including particular immune system actions at the entry points of infection, such as mouth or nose, and the way the system copes with the inflammations that result as the disease preliminarily makes inroads. Immunization short-circuits both the first stages of disease (the symptoms) and— and this may *seem* beneficial—the full mobilization of a person's immunity, which is definitely not helpful. It is because immunization evokes a *one-sided* mobilization of the body's defense that we will end up having to question vaccines' fundamental *raison d'être*. Before coming to that point, though, we will review equally serious, but less basic problems with immunization.

We will begin with (1) a survey of current immunization projects, with special attention to the government's recent broaching of the idea of mass smallpox immunizations. Then (2) we look at the history of immunizations, evaluating whether vaccines played the major role in ending epidemic disease claimed for them. Here we pay special attentions to smallpox vaccinations, which were the first in the field and have been championed as one of medicine's greatest triumphs. Next we look at adverse reactions that have been connected to the giving of inoculation, first (3) investigating those linked to additives (and contaminants); then (4) seeing about those charged to the vaccines proper. From there, we move on to considerations on what appear as questionable areas in vaccines' method of operation, looking at (5) whether DNA material from the decommissioned pathogens present in vaccines is able to work its way into our genetic software, and at (6) if early vaccine stimulation of our immune system possibly biases it toward the humoral branch of immune function. We move, finally, to social issues, (7) noting whether there has ever been hanky-panky in the promotion of vaccines—a look at the early days of polio will be of value here—and (8) seeing how those who have tried to opt out of the vaccination merry-go-round have suffered legal and medical persecution. We then discuss (9) necessary changes and (10) artificially versus naturally boosted immunity.

IMMUNIZATION TODAY AND TOMORROW: THE SMALLPOX VACCINE AND OTHER CANDIDATES FOR MASS IMMUNIZATION

Let us take for a moment the viewpoint of a Cynic, one of the early Greek philosophers who purported to see nothing but ulterior motives and thinly veiled egotism in all the actions of humans.[69] How would he look at the recent calls on the national level for the institutions of widespread inoculation of citizens with smallpox vaccine as a way to prepare the United States for a terrorist attack? This first step in our analysis is a thought experiment. In other words, I am not putting it forward as a serious proposal but as a way of opening our look into the entwining of hard science, prejudice, money, and publicity in our current commercial medical establishment.

We know that vaccine production is big business. Merck & Co., for example, rakes in $900 million a year on vaccine sales. It's no wonder that, as we document below, manufacturers are clamoring for the introduction of a smorgasbord of new vaccines. Pharmaceutical firms make plenty from these vaccines, and seldom do these immune cash cows run dry. But it can happen.

This came about in a celebrated way with smallpox. In 1977, WHO proclaimed the end of the disease. There was no variola virus, which causes the disease, existent upon the planet except in the high-security biowarfare facilities of Russia and the United States. The wiping out of this scourge was the sign for mass jubilation that reached from everyday people to white-coated scientists.

Perhaps the only place celebration was not heard, the Cynic would say, was in the laboratories of the smallpox vaccine makers. There the Cynic claimed to hear gnashing of teeth. "After all," we can imagine our Greek friend saying, "how can Vaccibucks Inc., with stocks of smallpox vaccine on hand and a vast plant primed to make more, ever use its capability now that the enemy it was geared up to fight has been totally expunged from the earth?"

The only hope for this pharmaceutical giant would be to find some ingenious way to convince people they had a dire need to take precautions against a disease that had been eliminated. Sound impossible? The cynic might tell the makers to look at the history of polio vaccine. In the United States, the last natural case of polio appeared in 1979. Yet more than twenty years later most school children are still mandated to take the vaccine. And this in the face of the fact that "the success of the international polio eradication efforts means that *the risk from oral [polio] vaccines is now greater than the risk posed by the disease.*"[70]

What justification has been used to keep up this seemingly irrational program? In a book by two pharmaceutical industry supporters, Margaret Hyde and Elizabeth Forsyth, this excuse is presented. "Many experts think such a step [discontinuing polio vaccination now that the disease has disappeared] would be foolish. Stocks of polio virus [used to make the vaccine] are now available globally, and there are concerns about accidental release, as well as the use of the virus by terrorists."[71]

Here's a real catch-22. We have to keep giving polio vaccinations because it's possible one of the many laboratory cultures of the disease will escape. But why do we need so many lab cultures of polio? *We need them to make the vaccine that will guard us against accidental release of polio from the vaccine-producing laboratories!*

To return to our parable, we might imagine the Cynic would say that to get people back to taking smallpox shots, its exponents would have to do no more than convince everyone there was a danger that terrorists would grab the virus from labs or that it would escape into the public through some other means.

We can end our thought experiment here. It departs from the truth in two ways. First, it is an overly dismissive view to believe not everyone would rejoice at the elimination of a disease, even those who might be hurt in the pocketbook by this medical victory. Second, it assumes the terrorist threat is not serious. Truthfully, the possibility of terrorists using smallpox as a bioweapon is credible, while, on the other hand, expectations that they would try to spread—the ideas of Hyde and Forsyth—polio are fantasy. Remember, smallpox is near the top of the CDC's list of likely biological warfare agents, while polio doesn't even appear on the comprehensive tally.

Still and all, there was a point to this exercise. It should make you realize that once the idea that smallpox may be used by terrorists was accepted, pharmaceutical interests would press for either immediate inoculation or the building of stockpiles of the vaccine, whether or not further revelations make it seem more or less probable that terrorists would use the variola virus in an onslaught.

Soon after the World Trade Center attack and the anthrax mailings, the federal health departments set to work to prepare for the advent of bioterrorists armed with smallpox virus. The first order of business was to build up supplies of the vaccine that could be used should smallpox appear. In June 2002, President Bush "signed into law a $4.6 billion bioterrorism prevention program, of which $640 million went to producing and stockpiling the smallpox vaccine."[72]

Although, as we will see, many doctors expressed dismay over the thought of inoculations with this vaccine, the government rushed ahead with plans to vaccinate those few people, such as medical personnel, who might be particularly vulnerable to the disease in case of terrorist attack. At the same time, tests of vaccine that had been frozen fifty years ago are in full swing.

The vaccine had been put in the deep freeze by Aventis Pasteur, a biological firm based in Swiftwater, Pennsylvania, thinking the military might need it. Now, the company has given 85 million doses to the United States government with the hopes that it is still usable. In order to try out the stock, a program was initiated in summer 2002, using three hundred paid volunteers from Oakland, California; Iowa City, Iowa; Nashville; and Houston to assess the quality of the medicine.

> During the testing in Oakland, nurses are injecting diluted versions of the Aventis vaccine in about forty to fifty people ages 18 to 32. Volunteers...will be paid $50 per visit and will keep a daily record of their physical symptoms, returning for periodic checkups and responding to follow-up telephone calls over the course of six months.[73]

Meanwhile, during the summer, conflicting reports appeared discussing what would be the best way to treat a terrorist smallpox episode, with opinions dividing between those who favor "ring vaccinations" and those who see more promise in blanket immunization. "Ring vaccinations" are those in which only those who have been in contact with an infected person are given shots, while blanket immunization involves inoculating whole communities where an outbreak has occurred.

Outside of the authors of a Yale study, not many favor blanket immunization. This study, made public July 8 by Edward Kaplan, principal investigator and a professor at the Yale University School of Management, argues that "vaccinating most or all of the population would make any post-attack strategy work better because fewer people would be vulnerable to the disease and fewer people would have to be given emergency vaccinations."[74]

Using a mathematical model of the spread of smallpox fomented by a terrorist action, Kaplan and associates compared the death rates of a ring vaccination versus a blanket vaccination strategies. "The model predicted mass vaccination would halt the spread of smallpox more rapidly and result in 4,120 fewer deaths in a city with 10 million inhabitants."[75] In Kaplan's view, while ring containment was an effective tactic in fighting Third World smallpox outbreaks—we will give details on this later—it cannot stand up to a terrorist onslaught. As he put it, "With a large scale attack, you're just not going to succeed in that endeavor."[76]

Other experts disagreed. Five advisers to the CDC, for example, came out saying that ring vaccination was the way to go. Dr. Lucy Tompkins, a Stanford University medical professor, spoke at a June 20 panel discussion on bioterrorist tactics. Tompkins and her fellow panelists agreed that inoculations should only be given "when an outbreak occurs. Even then, they argued that vaccinations should be given only to people who will come in contact with the infected."[77]

A recognition that the vaccine is liable to devastating side effects is what has dampened enthusiasm for immediate widespread inoculations. A piece by Keith Bradsher in the *New York Times* notes, "The vaccines had a high rate of side effects before their civilian use ended in 1972. Doctors predict that inoculating every American now would kill hundreds of people and leave another one thousand or more with brain damage."[78] This degree of adverse reactions is higher than that of any vaccine currently administered.

Dr. Richard P. Wenzel, chairman of MCV's Department of Internal Medicine, substantiates this claim by citing a 1970 study by Lane et al. of adverse reactions to the vaccine, which

> showed that for every 1 million Americans who received their
> first dose of vaccine, 242 developed a generalized vaccine-

related viral infection; 39 with pre-existing eczema developed a serious viral infection of their dermatitis...and 12
developed a life-threatening vaccine-related inflammation
of the brain (post-vaccine encephalitis). Thus, if we vaccinated just over one-third of our population, 100 million, we
could expect 1,200 cases of post-vaccine encephalitis. Possibly 100 to 300 would die as a result, and many others
would be left with neurological dysfunction.[79]

These are the stronger reactions, but almost equally disturbing is the
high rate of minor health detriments attributable to the vaccine. "Sore arms,
swollen lymph nodes and fever can occur in up to 50 percent of recipi-
ents."[80]

We can explain the unusually great number of side effects attributable
to smallpox vaccine to the fact that it makes uses of an actual live virus. Most
vaccines gain effectiveness by employing a weakened version of the targeted
pathogen in their preparations. The smallpox vaccine, in contrast, uses a full
potency cousin virus to smallpox to elicit the immune response. Because
this cousin virus, called vaccinia, "is live, it can spread to cause severe skin
infections, sometimes destroying tissue and causing permanent disability.
Or vaccinia can be spread just to the eye and permanently blind," as well as
causing encephalitis and the other dire conditions mentioned.[81]

Moreover, as Dr. John F. Modlin, chief of pediatrics at Dartmouth Medical School, points out, the extent of bad reactions to the vaccine can be expected to be higher now than they were when it was originally given since
there are many more Americans around with compromised immune systems. He told a *Washington Post* reporter, "Thirty and forty years ago, we
weren't treating patients with leukemia. we weren't doing kidney and liver
transplants, we didn't have HIV infections."[82] Persons with such weakened
constitutions have a higher probability of registering detrimental reactions
to the inoculation.

The proposal to simply give the vaccine to hospital personnel has also
been found objectionable, although many do consider this limited vaccination program as posing an acceptable risk. However, D. A. Henderson, head
of the Department of Health and Human Services (HHS) bioterrorism advisory
committee, disagrees. He says, "Trying to vaccinate your health care workers
in advance—we don't think it's a good idea."[83] He doesn't like the thought of
even limited vaccination because of the danger of disease shedding.

"Shedding" takes place when a vaccinated patient passes the disease he
or she has been inoculated with, in this case vaccinia, to an unvaccinated

person. Dr. Julie Gerberding, acting deputy director of the CDC, explains, "If you get immunized with vaccinia, you can infect people around you from your vaccinia scab. So while you may accept the risk for yourself, you would be imparting a risk to your contacts."[84]

All these problems with the vaccine are compounded by shortfalls on what should be known by physicians and available as palliatives. To deal with the second point first, there is a natural substance, vaccine immune globulin, which can be given to those who are suffering ill effects from the vaccine. However, while there are millions of doses of the vaccine ready to use and more on the way, vaccine immune globulin is in short supply. There is only enough of the substance to treat about six hundred patients![85]

Furthermore, confidence in the results of any kind of smallpox inoculation campaign is certainly not buoyed up by the findings of a recent survey, which indicated United States physicians are blithely unaware of any dangers associated with the vaccine. The survey was commissioned by the CDC and entailed one-hour interviews with doctors from Philadelphia, Chicago, and San Francisco. The findings were made public on May 9, 2002. "The interviews revealed that many doctors mistakenly believe smallpox vaccine is as safe as common childhood vaccines, such as measles shots."[86] On top of that, younger doctors are misinformed about the current prevalence of the disease as well as how to treat it. "Most doctors, particularly those under age forty, do not know how to use the two-pronged needle required to administer the vaccine, the survey found."[87]

Given this generalized ignorance, it would seem even a partial immunization program should be preceded by a thoroughgoing education about the disease and its treatment Otherwise, according to Robert Daum, a pediatric infectious disease specialist at the University of Chicago, "What might be spread is not just smallpox, but terror."[88]

Worries about these disadvantages of the vaccine have spread all the way to the top of the world medical hierarchy. The director-general of WHO, Dr. Gro Brundtland, has already spoken out against using the vaccine wholesale. On October 26, 2001, he said, "Existing vaccines have proven efficacy but also have a high incidence of adverse side-effects. The risk of adverse events is sufficiently high that mass vaccination is not warranted if there is no or little risk of exposure."[89]

Putting aside pure and simple health issues, we can add that this vaccine has been bothered, though to a lesser extent, with the same accusations of financial favoritism that we saw plaguing anthrax vaccine production.

The *Washington Post* featured a story on the claims of three small companies who charged they were not let into the running on government contracts to produce smallpox vaccine. These companies "have done considerable work on smallpox vaccines over the last two years," and say they could lease space for mass production.[90]

In selecting finalists, HHS put aside the proven capability as a selection criterion in favor of girth. Two of the three mega-pharmaceutical firms selected, namely, Merck and GlaxoSmithKline, "have done little work in recent decades on smallpox vaccines, but have their own big laboratories."[91] Moreover, where the bids of the small companies hit the government target of $2 a dose, the finalists bids "were much higher than anticipated," and above the asked-for price.

Because drugs cost so much, the HHS has come up with an inventive solution. "Health officials hope to stretch the existing stock of fifteen million doses of the old vaccine by diluting it."[92] Anthony Fauci, head of HHS, stated that preliminary tests showed that even when given at one tenth strength the vaccine is still 70 percent effective.

The obvious question is: Is the watered-down vaccine really effective or is it being touted because it will save money? There is also a less obvious question: Granted that the smallpox vaccine has a record of unusually high adverse reactions, and that such reactions are less drastic, the smaller the dose, why had previous smallpox eradication campaigns utilized such a dangerously potent amount?

These last few paragraphs have gotten away from our central theme, the value and drawbacks of the vaccine, but they were included to keep us aware of the edge of self interest that enters into many decisions that have been and are being made about vaccines. The HHS doesn't want to scare the public by presenting it with too large a bill for anti-terrorism measures, and so looks to cut costs. The small drug companies want a slice of the action, while the big ones, who had long cultivated cosy contracts with government health officials, rush to bid for a contract on a vaccine they have had little previous interest in. If these firms didn't hold every big money contract the government offered, their monopoly positions would be in jeopardy.

Similar examples of self interest can be found if we turn away from vaccines being created at the moment to see which ones are on the drawing board. James Odell, writing in the *Townsend Letter for Doctors and Patients* in January 2002, scouted new vaccine initiatives being proposed by the Institute of Medicine (IOM).

He notes, in passing, that the IOM, a division of the National Academy of Sciences, which advises the government on which vaccine developments should be funded, is hardly as free from influence peddling as an scientific agency should be. "Its corporate donor list reads like a *Who's Who* of the medical industrial complex," featuring such names as Monsanto, the AMA, blood bank trade associations, the March of Dimes.[93] Members of the IOM committees are frequently executives from pharmaceutical companies, and this to such a degree the *Scientific American* was outraged. The journal editorialized that it had serious concerns about the objectivity of the division in light of its "cozy relationship with external parties."[94]

It's no surprise, then, that the Institute of Medicine tends to back proposals for vaccines favored by major pharmaceutical firms. (The IOM has an excellent track record as far as seeing the vaccines it backs get commissioned, created, and put into circulation. For example, six of the fourteen vaccines it sponsored in 1984 have been licensed and in some area mandated for school children.) It's even less a surprise that the IOM rallied behind a measure that would shift liability for injuries linked to inoculations to the federal government and away from the vaccine manufacturers. A particular vaccine might only benefit one maker, but this law would redound to the advantage of all the big drug firms. In 1985, the institute issued a report that suggested "political decision makers develop a compensation system for vaccine-related injury."[95] Subsequently, such a law was put into effect and now the government assumes costs for damages awarded those injured by vaccines, which has proven "a huge financial benefit for vaccine manufacturers," who, of course, now have "little incentive to improve existing products," since they won't have to pay for any injury their vaccines may cause.[96]

And don't think these vaccine producers don't know which side their bread is buttered on. In Congressional testimony, a vaccine maker admitted his company made a hefty contribution to the IOM to support its 1985 pro-industry study.

So what is the IOM recommending now? A 1999 report outlining priorities for the coming twenty years stressed vaccines that would be used against sexually transmitted diseases, including AIDS, influenza, and even…drug addiction!

The National Academy division saw as "most favorable" the prospects for creating vaccines against the STDs: chlamydia, herpes, human pappillomavirus, and gonorrhea. Once these are ready to go, Odell italicizes, "*these are specified for administration to all 12-year-olds.*"[97]

The AIDS vaccine is another biggie, though, as we have discussed elsewhere, every attempt to create such a inoculation has so far been an abject failure, perhaps because no one has a very clear idea of what the vaccine's target, HIV, looks like.[98]

The nasal flu vaccine is the closest of these drugs to licensing, being about two years down the road. It is expected to be mandated for administration to all school children, its backers hoping it won't be as ineffective as other flu vaccines already in use.

Last in the docket of vaccines being researched is that which would guard against cocaine addiction. This flies under the rather dubious and unproven assumption that drug addiction is caused by or closely akin to an infectious disease. However, it would certainly be profitable to pharmaceutical companies if drug abuse seemed to demand a high-priced pill or shot as something that would end craving. Moreover the current vaccine would not be given only to active abusers. Peter Cohen of the National Institute of Drug Abuse, part of the NIH, "suggested giving a future cocaine addiction vaccine to all children, so that cocaine addicts are not stigmatized."[99]

THE CHECKERED HISTORY OF IMMUNIZATION

Now that we have depicted some of the controversy swirling around the question of whether national smallpox immunization should be rolled out as a defense against bioterrorist action, it might be appropriate to look into the history of smallpox vaccinations since this is hardly the first time the vaccine has been the focus of debate. Here we can also make some broader observations about the place of medicine in disease control.

Earlier we referred to the glorious day of May 8, 1980, when the World Health Organization declared the dread disease of smallpox expunged from the earth. Perhaps, there is an extra poignancy to the fact that the smallpox vaccine was the first ever developed. It was experimented with in the late 1700s by the Dr. Edward Jenner of Britain who created it using material from people infected with cowpox, hence the name "vaccine" from the Latin "vacca" or cow. It seems the vaccine that was first on the field was the first one to totally eliminate its disease adversary.

The glowing story of Jenner's "discovery" of vaccinations has been told and retold, warts and all. I put "discovery" in quotes in that similar methods of inoculation had been used for centuries in the East. Donald Henderson from John Hopkins and Bernard Moss of the NIH date the appearance of vaccination to AD 1000 in India. "From India, the practice spread to China, Western Asia, and Africa, and finally, in the early eighteenth century, to Europe and North America."[100] It reached England through the good offices of Lady Mary Wortley Montagu, who proselytized for a method of vaccination she had seen practiced in Turkey. There pus from smallpox sores was inserted in an inoculee's arm by needle.[101] Jenner built on an understanding of prevention garnered from folk culture. Where he advanced beyond former knowledge was in drawing the pus from milkmaids affected with cowpox, which he guessed was a disease from the same family as smallpox, though it was not as nasty a customer.

The stories are narrated, I say, "warts and all," in that they often portray Jenner's lack of experimental ethics. Hyde and Forsyth, great defenders of vaccination, do not whitewash this aspect of the story. "Jenner selected a healthy eight-year-old boy named James Phipps, for a human experiment.... [After previously inoculating him with cowpox pus] He scratched some human smallpox pus under the boy's skin." The boy didn't have much say in the matter. He was lucky; the experiment turned out well. As Hyde and Forsyth state, "Jenner's experiment would not be permitted today. In Jenner's time, however, there were no committees on medical ethics."[102]

Jenner skated around these ethical questions and was successful in getting money from Parliament for mass inoculations in 1802 and 1807. The only place his program didn't go as planned was in preventing disease. Not only was he blocked by religious groups and ethical societies "who opposed the principle of infecting humans with an animal disease," but his own vaccine often misfired.[103] "Confidence in the [cowpox inoculation] procedure was also diminished by the occurrence of smallpox in some who previously had been successfully vaccinated. Jenner had forcefully contended that protection was lifelong."[104]

At the time, and for decades after, it was not recognized that the cowpox vaccination, though it gave short-term protection against the virus, did not offer the type of long-term immunity that one would obtain from actually surviving the disease. Because the necessity for booster shots (later doses of a particular type of inoculation one has already taken in order to renew the waning protection of the first dose) was not yet grasped; smallpox deaths in England (where the vaccination program originated and was most extensive) continued to be racked up even as a larger and larger percentage of the population got their shots.

Compulsory vaccination in Britain really began in 1852. From 1857 to 1859, 14,244 still died from smallpox. Even in 1872, after a inoculation drive saw 97 percent of the population vaccinated, "England experienced its worst-ever smallpox vaccination: 44,840 lives were lost."[105]

The situation was not helped in the beginning by the way vaccination advocates, rather than recognizing the insufficiencies of their vaccine, blamed everything else. According to Neil Miller,

> Jenner [and his followers] said anyone coming down with
> smallpox after vaccination wasn't taking the formula made
> to his specifications. So they called it spurious cowpox.
> Then they started blaming improperly administered injec-
> tions.[106]

Henderson and Moss argue that the development of booster shots and other improvements created a viable anti-smallpox measure, which would eventually prove its worth when administered worldwide in the WHO battle to stamp out the disease. (We may note that Miller disputes whether the vaccine was ever very effective.)

The two refinements Henderson and Moss mention as perfecting the preparation are a change in production, so that instead of cowpox taken from the pails of milkmaids, smallpox was taken from infected calves and then weakened; and, in the 1940s, the creation of "a commercially feasible process for the large-scale production of a stable freeze-dried vaccine."[107] Having a freeze-dryable product disposed of the problem of transporting the vaccine and keeping it fresh in underdeveloped lands. Till this development, it would have been impossible to carry out viable disease elimination in countries that were far from the labs where the vaccine was produced and that lacked widespread refrigeration.

Although we don't have the evidence to pass judgment on exactly how effective the smallpox vaccine is, there are two points that should be made up front, before we look at broader patterns of disease fluctuation. These points should temper our enthusiasm for the achievement of vaccination, though they hardly dispute that it has been of great service to humankind.

The first fact relates to the inaugural campaign to curtail smallpox in England. Boosters such as Hyde and Forsyth wax eloquent about how "as the number of people who received vaccinations increased, the number of cases of smallpox decreased."[108] They trumpet that smallpox was quickly wiped out in Britain and other Western countries.

Smallpox did decrease precipitously in England, but what vaccine proponents tend to downplay is the fact that smallpox was not a very prominent disease in the West at the time of its decline. For instance, in England, and making a comparison only with other airborne infections, McKeown writes, "In 1848–54, the death rate from the disease was only 263 (per million), less than a tenth of the rate for respiratory tuberculosis and considerably lower than the rates from whooping cough and measles."[109] It was not a major killer then, though its declension did mark a significant improvement in national health.

Turning to the global crusade, I want to note something that doesn't touch on vaccinations per se but on the significance of mass inoculations. It's a point we've already seen raised in discussing the stormy battle over whether to reinstitute smallpox vaccinations in the United States.

One would think from reading the texts coming from the pro-vaccine camp that to wipe out smallpox WHO simply inoculated everyone in the Third World. However, scholars have argued that it was not mass vaccination but the quick identification of people with the disease, and then these patients' isolation, coupled with the inoculation of their immediate contacts that won the battle. In other words, what did the trick was ring vaccination.

> This conclusion is supported by experience in India, where smallpox remained a serious problem in spite of a mass vaccination until adequate surveillance and containment were introduced. Similarly, in the very successful West African programme, smallpox was eradicated, without achieving a high level of immunity in the population, by concentrating on case detection, outbreak investigation and vaccination of contacts. Again, the 1972 Khulna epidemic in Bangladesh was brought rapidly under control through selective immunization of high risk groups; mass vaccination was not undertaken and the general level of immunity in the population is believed to have remained essentially the same.[110]

As we've seen, the debate over the effectiveness of ring vaccinations is still ongoing. I would venture to say that the role targeted vaccinations took in overcoming smallpox worldwide is downplayed by immunization proponents, because they are trying to align past triumphs with what they defend in the present. Grasping how a particular infectious disease was stopped in the past is important to understanding of how to proceed against pathogens today. And, there is an even greater historical issue in the wings. Beyond interrogating history to find out which methods seem significant in elimination of a single sickness, one can ratchet this up a bit, and ask further what medical methods, if any, played a part in the larger rhythms of epidemic fluctuation.

At this juncture, we want to provide a broader historical canvas so as to assess the relationship between humans and germs over the centuries. We will proceed in two stages. First, we look at the accommodation worked out over the centuries between these two competitive groups, and, second, we will investigate the near total elimination of infectious disease in the West in the last century and a half, asking why it came about.

If we turn back to prehistory when hunters and gatherers roamed the earth in small bands, the best estimates we have is that, while life may have been short due to starvation or injury from wild beasts, infectious illness was not a big problem.

> During most of his existence man has been a comparatively rare animal living in small groups of no more than a few hundred persons. Such conditions do not permit transmission and survival of many micro-organisms, and some years ago Burnet suggested that infectious diseases as we now know them did not exist.[111]

The coming of such diseases would have to wait for the larger density of populations found with agriculture. "Many infections require minimal host populations if they are to be maintained, and it is only after the first agricultural revolution that human populations reached the size needed for the perpetuation of many organisms that have no animal host."[112] Moreover, once humans lived in small, immobile communities, they became a magnet for rats, flies, and other insects and small animals that served as disease reservoirs. Of even more importance for the generation of disease was that in these communities people began raising domestic livestock. "Most and probably all of the distinctive infectious diseases of civilization transferred to human populations from animal herds."[113]

As we explained earlier, once these diseases got going, they tended to move toward less virulent forms, while through natural selection humans became more resistant. Certainly, natural selection is a harsh way to get around disease by improving human stock. People who are not resistant to an illness are killed off, leaving the less susceptible to reproduce.

Simple natural selection, by the way, also can be used to account for the de-virulization of germs. The case of myxomatosis and the Australian rabbit is often cited in this context. European colonists introduced rabbits into Australia where the animals ran wild and got out of control. Then the colonists, in order to clean up the mess, infected rabbits with the myxomatosis virus, which is spread by mosquito. The virus started off with a 99 percent mortality rate, however, within a few years, less murderous strains appeared, and mortality decreased. C. Andrewes explains why this friendlier virus quickly out-proliferated the more potent type. "A less vicious virus permitted the rabbit to live longer; it was thus available for a longer time as a source of virus for biting mosquitoes, and thus was spread more widely."[114]

McNeill goes to great pains to show how isolated human groups, infected and reinfected with the same diseases, ended up learning to live with the germs, which, in return, became producers of less serious illness. The historian emphasize that the great plagues of the last five hundred years, such as the measles and smallpox that nearly exterminated the American Indians when they were infected by Europeans, have always been found to occur when a new pathogen is introduced into an inexperienced community.

We can say that once transportation linkages had tied the earth together, there was a gradual lessening of the impact of most infectious diseases. "On the time scale of world history," McNeill writes, "we should view the 'domestication' of epidemic disease that occurred between AD 1300 and AD 1700 as a fundamental breakthrough directly resulting from the two great transportation revolutions of that age."[115] He continues,

> There emerged a new relation between humankind and the parasitic micro-organisms. It was a more stable pattern of parasitism, less destructive to human hosts, and correspondingly more secure for the parasites. The infectious organism could count on a fresh supply of susceptible children, whose numbers and availability were subject to far less statistical variation than had been the case when epidemic patterns of disease had produced alternate feast and famine for the organisms infecting humanity. Both sides were more secure and in that sense better off.[116]

Lest this seem to present too rosy a picture, let us keep in mind that this uneasy coexistence between human and microparasite, though it precluded epidemic, did entail very large infant mortality rates, with half or more newborns succumbing to illness. So far this history of the interadaptation of microbes and humans suggests two conclusions.

The first is that no matter how much more humanitarian the use of vaccines is as compared to the Darwinian method, it does have an obvious downside. With the use of vaccines, we will never develop the live-and-let-live attitude that earlier generations gained. Instead of interacting with specific germs until they become relatively benign, we don't allow our immune systems to meet them unaided. The germs come into the human body where they are beset by antibiotics, antivirals, or primed antibodies, and so the microbes evolve toward greater skill at escaping destruction. They move toward more not less antagonism.

This is a small price to pay, it could be said, since we seem, by way of vaccines, to have escaped the ravages of so many debilitating sicknesses. However, a second, more disquieting thought is this. We are seeing that over centuries humans physiologically found ways to withstand illness. The Darwinian one can probably safely be left behind, but what about the complex activities of the immune system. Are some of these being undercut as the way to handle infections is displaced from our bodies to our medicine chests? This is a topic we will take up shortly.

However, the foregoing implies that the advent of vaccines and other infection-stanching drugs fundamentally altered the tug of war between pathogens and humans. Certainly, that is a widely received idea, but a closer scrutiny of the historical record, as has been carried out by Richard McKeown in his *The Modern Rise of Population* may teach us otherwise.

McKeown's meticulous examination of British death notices established the following startling fact. When he sought the reasons for the spectacular fall of illness-produced mortality from the nineteenth century on, he found out that not only vaccinations but medicine itself played a *trivial* role.

To give some figures so that what I'm talking about is clear, I refer to a chart in McKeown's book (not reproduced here) on measles mortality data for children. In 1890, deaths were about 1,200 per million, while in 1935, they were about 100 per million.[117] So by 1934, measles deaths had fallen 1,200 percent from what they had been forty years earlier.

What did medicine have to do with this? In 1935, a useful chemotherapy to combat secondary infections associated with the disease appeared. This was the first medical procedure invented to lessen measles' impact. Vaccines didn't come on the scene till the 1960s.

The point is representative. Measles had disappeared as a serious health threat by the time any medical headway against it had been made.

A worse killer, respiratory tuberculosis, saw an equally sharp drop, from a death rate in 1838 of four thousand per million to one, in 1940, of about four hundred per million.[118] For TB, effective treatment began to be used in 1947, again, after its mortality rate had dropped to one tenth of what it had been one hundred years earlier.

(Smallpox is the only anomaly here, since vaccinations did help temper its impact. However, as noted before, smallpox was not the major killer that measles and TB were.)

So why did these diseases virtually disappear before medicine found any treatments against them?

It was not, as one might guess from reading McNeill, that the microbes had all simultaneously evolved into more beneficent forms. Their potency was undiminished.

Some might think that the central role must have gone to public health improvements, such as the provision of clean water, good sewage and garbage disposal, and untampered-with food. By lessening human's contact with pathogens, these reform lessened the inroads against diseases, such as cholera, that were spread through food, waste, and water. But such improvements had minimal effects on the major killers, such as tuberculosis, which moved through the air, spread by a sick person's coughing or via contaminated dust.

What lowered the impact of this group of infections is something often overlooked: adequate food for the impoverished majority. For McKeown, given that the airborne killers, which were not affected by public health measures, led in deaths, better nutrition is far and away the primary reason for the decline in disease-related mortality.

> In Europe there was a large increase in food supplies be-
> tween the end of the seventeenth century and the mid-
> nineteenth, in Britain sufficient to feed a population that
> had trebled in size, without significant imported food. This
> increase coincided with a substantial reduction of mortal-
> ity from infectious disease and, it is suggested, was the
> main reason for it.[119]

Medical studies, McKeown goes on, have shown a intimate connection between malnutrition/under-nutrition and the contraction of infections. In underdeveloped countries, it has been found "malnutrition contributes largely to the high levels of infectious deaths."[120]

Looking even further back from the period we are concerned with, McKeown supplements the work of McNeill with his own thoughts about the appearance of infections. Remember, McNeill hypothesized that human infectious diseases appeared when the settled life of agriculturalists and pastoralists created a large pool of infectable people. McKeown adds to this picture. "It was critical to this relationship [that between germ and human being] that it evolved over a period when the human host was, in general, poorly nourished."[121]

You may complain we have strayed far from the topic of the history of vaccines, but hold your fire a minute. We just mentioned that studies of conditions in the Third World have found a close correlation between infectious disease and malnutrition. So, we might ask: How does this information sit in relation to attempts to control diseases, such as smallpox, in underdeveloped countries?

A spokesman for the World Health Organization states that giving medicine to a half-starved people is fruitless. "It is questionable whether infectious disease can be controlled by vaccination in undernourished populations.[122] A different writer, also a WHO spokesperson and also discussing the situation in underdeveloped regions, puts this thought even more strongly. "For the time being...an adequate diet is the most effective '*vaccine*' against most of the diarrhoeal, respiratory and other common infections [found in these countries]."[123]

This is certainly relevant to plans being put forward, such as those who are concerned with AIDS in Africa, to use vaccines and other drugs to solve the problem. But this doesn't seem to touch on the situation in America. We need to see that McKeown's viewpoint is derived from the new medical paradigm, which he identifies in this manner:

> The health of man is determined essentially by his behaviour, his food and the nature of the world around him, and is only marginally influenced by personal medical care. Intuitively we believe that *we are ill and made well*, it is nearer the truth to say that we *are well and are made ill*. [124]

Here is an analogy that's more than analogy. If it's true that more plentiful, better food, rather than vaccines and medical care, is responsible for the near abolishment of the epidemic diseases of the nineteenth century, is it also possible that for us in the United States our best chance against the new germs invading our ecosphere, even those used by terrorists, will be through improving our nutrition. For if our ancestors and people in the underdeveloped world lack full nutrition because of the unavailability of food, we seem to lack it because our foods have been industrially stripped of nutrients. We need to consider what we can do to optimize our health though avoidance of such foods and practice detoxification to rid ourselves of their effects.

Before we take up this topic in earnest, let's move from a study of vaccines' past to their present and see if any now on the market are still as culpable as Jenner's first overly promoted, unimproved anti-pox.

ADVERSE REACTIONS TO VACCINES: ADDITIVES

To be clear at outset, in discussing vaccines and toxicities, our purpose is not to issue a blanket condemnation of immunization, but to sift through scientific studies that note suggestive links between the administration of a vaccine and the onset of enfeebling symptoms. It may well be, as we will show later, that a round of almost any vaccine will detrimentally over-develop one part of the immune system. This criticism would find all vaccines culpable. However, at this point, what we are going to do is note the specific adverse results that appear in tandem with particular vaccines given in particular sequences.

In going through these materials, we need to keep in mind that what research we have is contradictory. Two studies that were published in the same year (1998) in the prestigious British medical journal, *Lancet*, illustrate this point. One by Andrew Wakefield and associates cited twelve cases that suggested a link between the MMR vaccine (Mumps-Measles-Rubella) and autism. A second piece by Brent Taylor, which was picked up and trumpeted by the vaccine industry, said there was no such connection.

At this stage, it is impossible to decide between such studies, although overall there are not a lot to choose from. This is the most scandalous feature of the whole situation. There is a crying need for studies of vaccines and their adverse (or lack of adverse) reactions, but they are not being done. When the IOM, which we have seen is not in any way prejudiced against vaccines, was asked in 1991 and 1994 to prepare reports for the government on vaccine safety, it confessed "There is very little data on vaccine safety because the necessary research is simply not being done."[125] Writing in March 1999, Philip Incao, MD, re-echoes this point and remarks further that the type of studies that are needed would be ones where a group of vaccinated children are juxtaposed to a group of unvaccinated children and each group's health is observed. "Incredible as it sounds," Incao remarks, "such a common-sense controlled study comparing vaccinated to unvaccinated children has never been done in America for any vaccine."[126]

It is doubtful whether such studies will be financed any time soon. The sad fact is that research depends on funding, and funding is most likely to come from government or pharmaceutical industry coffers. You only have to look at the decades of neglect of the question of the relation between smoking and lung cancer (while billions were poured into unrelated cancer research) to see the warped priorities of our research commissioning system. Funding tends to go to those who keep their hands off touchy subjects.

The type of evidence we are going to survey as we dip into the topic of adverse reactions is mainly correlative. Two forms of correlation will be stressed. One is that which notes a temporal sequence in which the appearance of a perverse health condition follows vaccination. This means that, to take an actual example, a child gets a pertussis (whooping cough) shot, feels sick, and ends with encephalitis, an inflammation that causes brain damage. A second kind of correlation ties the introduction a particular immunization to the appearance or increase of a particular debilitating state. Here, we put, for example, the finding of Dr. Bernard Rimland, which was that "a sharp rises in the incidence of autism in the U.S.A. took place immediately following the introduction of the MMR vaccine in 1975, and in the United Kingdom following its introduction in 1988."[127]

Bear in mind, *correlation cannot take the place of proof.* The materials we are examining do not prove the vaccine is responsible for the condition that followed. This is a point we hammer on in our in our AIDS book. There we note that a central dilemma for those who push the doctrine HIV = AIDS is that, though they have shown to their own satisfaction that HIV exists in all people with AIDS, they haven't been able to isolate HIV and transfer it to a cell culture or animal subject to see whether it would cause that culture or animal to experience AIDS. But if they have not done this, they have not shown a direct cause and effect relationship between the retrovirus and the disease. Simply finding the two in bed together, as it were, that is, finding a disease and a new microbe co-present, is not satisfactory proof. Both may have been caused by a third pathogen. Or the microbe may be a co-factor, needed but not sufficient by itself to bring on the disease state.

We don't want to follow these HIV = AIDS advocates, who often act as if correlation alone is enough evidence to verify their point. However, we must stress that those vaccine defenders who contemptuously dismiss such correlations—as when Hyde and Forsythe state that those who see a link between the giving of a DTP (diptheria/tetanus/pertussis) vaccination to an infant and that infant's death from SIDS (sudden infant death syndrome) as an "example of mistaken reasoning"—seem overly complacent.[128]

"Just by chance alone," Hyde and Forsyth write, "a certain number of deaths could be expected to occur after immunization."[129] True enough, but the disturbing facts are that SIDS increased as vaccine use increased and that SIDS has no known cause. Certainly, vaccines should be one suspect, if not the only one, in our investigation of this terrifying new killer.

Lest we go too far in making our claims seem speculative, it should be mentioned that there are some adverse reactions to vaccines that everyone acknowledges. Recall the case of Tom Colosimo, the soldier whose health broke down after he was vaccinated with anti-anthrax formulas. Speaking for the military, Marine Major General Randall West said Colosimo's physical deterioration was due to his immunizations. So the question at issue is not whether vaccines can cause damage, it is: How frequently do cases of this damage occur? The industry says such ill effects are found extremely rarely; vaccine opponents say they are common enough with some vaccines to call for a moratorium on their use.

In such circumstances, the least we can say is that in relation to those vaccines with the worst records, one should proceed with extreme caution. It is highly questionable whether infants with their not-yet-fully-operational immune systems should be burdened with weakened disease germs conveyed to them in vaccines. Further, pharmaceutical companies themselves admit it is unsafe to give an inoculation to someone with compromised immunity.

Let us begin our investigation by looking to the hazardous nature of certain vaccine additives, drawing on the book *Vaccination Roulette*, published by the Australian Vaccination Network (AVN) in 1998.

We mentioned earlier that it is not possible simply to shoot a weakened virus or bacterium into someone's veins. "Each vaccine has its own preservative, neutralizer, and carrying agent."[130] The AVN has tried to assess whether these additives have ill effects. They do not try to link specific additives to particular reactions to immunization, which would be an extremely difficult task insofar as it would demand separating out the body's reaction to one element in a mixture from reaction to the whole mixture. What the authors concentrate on is how specific additives, those being phenol, formaldehyde, and thiomersal, have been implicated as promoters of disease or allergic reaction when used on their own.

Folk wisdom accords with critical science in this context, since once the public knows what a particular substance is used for in other contexts—that formaldehyde is used for embalming, for instance—it wants nothing to do with it. And the public holds this position despite the empty assurances of vaccine advocates who write, for example, "Although mercury can be poisonous, the small amount of thiomersal [a mercury compound] that is added to vaccines contains very little mercury, and there is no evidence that it has caused harm."[131]

We will look at these three additives in turn, beginning each discussion with a notation on what other uses have been found for the additive outside of its being used in vaccines.

PHENOL

This chemical, also known as carbolic acid, was once used as an antiseptic but was later discontinued in that role because less corrosive disinfectants were discovered. It is a major component in creosote, the tarry substance put on railroad ties to prevent them from rotting.

We know that the swallowing of "as little as one gram can be fatal to humans."[132] This swallowing would cause a burning sensation in the mouth and throat. Penetrating to the brain, the drug, depending on the dosage, can cause seizures, coma, and an interference with control of the heart's rhythm.

FORMALDEHYDE

This chemical, as noted, is necessary for embalming as well as in the manufacture of particular car parts, furniture, and carpets.

Formaldehyde is a prominent allergen (allergic reaction inducer), affecting perhaps a fifth of the United States population. Exposure to formaldehyde can bring on nose bleeds, nausea, irritation of the eyes, nose, and throat, among other reactions. The EPA has listed it as a probable human carcinogen. "According to chemistry and toxicology books, formaldehyde should NEVER be injected into live tissues."[133] Further, even minuscule amounts will trigger a dangerous response in those who are allergic to it.

THIOMERSAL

This substance is a compound of mercury. Mercury, well known from its use in thermometers, is used both to dissolve and amalgamate other metals. For instance, as a solvent, it is used to release gold from the ore it is found in. As an amalgam, it is found in the mercury fillings used in traditional dentistry, where it joins the silver, zinc, copper and other metals in the tooth replacement.

Many of you may also be aware of the problems these fillings cause as the mercury leeches out of them into the mouth. In *Get Healthy Now*, I give some details on the health problems associated with this leakage. Mercury interferes with enzymes in the cells by substituting for the zinc that is used in the their production. This can cause numerous problems. "The most common symptoms of mercury toxicity are fatigue, depression, inability to concentrate, memory deficit, gastrointestinal tract problems, kidney problems, and frequent infections."[134]

Thiomersal itself has been tied in with a number of health problems, particularly to those who are sensitive to the chemical. These problems include headache, nausea, and vomiting. In June 1999, the Food and Drug Administration concluded that "infants who receive thimerosal [thiomersal] injections may be exposed to more mercury than recommended by Federal guidelines for total mercury exposure."[135]

Aside from these chemical additives, various vaccines contain biological substances, such as ones drawn from calf serum, chick embryos, and monkey kidney cells "These foreign proteins…are potential allergens and can produce anaphylactic shock [a severe and possibly fatal reaction to an allergen]."[136]

Pharmaceutical companies themselves have recognized the problematic character of some of the additives they are employing and are working to find substitutes. For one, "vaccine makers are working to eliminate or reduce the use of thiomersol."[137]

Aside from the health hazards that may occur in relation to provocations given by the additives purposefully included with the vaccine, there are those difficulties that may be stirred up by unintentional additives, that is, contaminants.

In January 2001, Dr. Harold Clark published a short note in the *Townsend Letter for Doctors* to report on some experiments done at his research institute testing commercially available vaccines for the presence of mycoplasmas. Mycoplasmas are types of parasitic microorganisms that are much smaller than bacteria and other cellular life forms. Some types of pneumonia and certain urinary tract infections are caused by these pathogens.

In 1956, when vaccines were first being developed, they were found to be laced with these tiny organisms. If the mycoplasmas in the contaminated vaccines were disease agents, then the vaccines would foster a rather paradoxical situation. A person would be injected with a weakened bacteria, say, on which, riding piggyback, was a strong disease agent, raring to go. The trouble was so bad that federal regulations concerning vaccine production were rewritten to insure that pharmaceutical firms paid attention to the danger. The relevant passage in the new law stated, "Only when the virus pool shows no evidence of Mycoplasmas is the viral pool considered acceptable for vaccine manufacture."[138]

This would seem to have corrected the problems, except that the regulation as well as the tests used for their presence of microorganisms were focused exclusively on whole mycoplasmas. The screening vaccine makers now carry out "does not exclude mycoplasma fragments or antigens."[139] Although importing these contaminants into the vaccine would not pose the same difficulty as that brought about by bringing in full-fledged microorganisms, it would, according to Clark, still introduce destabilizing influences in the body. He argues that the antigens of the mycoplasmas can interfere with the human immune system and initiate "pathogenicity."[140]

That such mycoplasmic detritus was not tested for does not mean that it was finding its way into vaccines. To see what the real state of affairs was vis-a-vis vaccines and mycoplasmas motivated the Mycoplasma Research Institute to examine commercial vaccines, looking at both the weakened viruses used to make some of them, such as those for polio and measles, as well as at the MMR vaccine itself. Among the findings were that "Polio type 1 virus was contaminated with 2 mycoplasma antigens"; while a rabbit given the MMR vaccine, who had been free of the tiny microorganisms prior to vaccination, showed evidence "of three of the eight mycoplasma strains tested" after the injection.[141] Though one study does not provide conclusive proof, it does indicate the strong possibility that mycoplasmas are fouling some vaccine preparations.

The piggyback paradox, whereby a vaccine is carrying not only a weakened pathogen but also (unknowingly) a potent one, has haunted vaccine makers from the beginning. In *AIDS: A Second Opinion*, we take up the case of the first developed polio vaccines, whose readily admitted contamination is not in question. We write there:

> The fact that one of the polio vaccines used in Africa was contaminated with a monkey virus has been abundantly acknowledged and verified. As Curtis describes, "There was, in fact, an almost forgotten mass vaccination campaign in which an oral polio vaccine was administered to at least 325,000 people, and perhaps more than half a million people, in equatorial Africa from 1957 to 1960."[142] Later it was found that one of the two vaccines used in the program was laced with monkey virus.
>
> When I say this contamination has been "acknowledged," I mean at the highest possible level. The revered developer of the vaccine, Jonas Salk, has confessed this was a tragic error, though one he feels is excusable. "We took all the precautions that we knew of at the time," Salk says, but "sometimes you find out things after the fact."[143] He goes on to talk about SV-40, the monkey virus, which…was mixed in with all the early vaccines. [Salk states:]
>
> SV40 virus…was a contaminant in monkey kidney cell cultures. The last thing in the world one would want to do

now is to make vaccines out of the tissues of monkeys that come from the jungle. That was a learning experience, you might say.[144]

In *AIDS*, we explain how human ignorance of the different animal viruses brought about this unfortunate situation.

> Polio virus is grown in primate cells. "Either monkey or human cells will work, but researchers selected monkeys because their tissue was more available and there were fears that human cell lines might spread cancer."[145] Specifically, in the 1950s, polio viruses were cultured on monkey kidneys.
>
> Some of these kidneys were infected with viruses. "Scientists knew about some of these viruses and developed tests to identify and then eliminate the tissues that contained them."[146] But, as we know now, at least one of these viruses, SV-40 (the fortieth monkey virus identified) evaded detection.
>
> Between 1954 and 1963, an estimated 10 million to 30 million Americans and scores of millions of people around the world were exposed to a virus that infected the kidneys of the Asian rhesus monkeys imported mainly from India. The virus survived the formaldehyde that Salk used to kill his polio viruses.[147]

Another recurrent pattern in the history of vaccines that we find in the story of polio's contamination is the paucity of research on what would seem to be a subject crying out for such handling. Curtis points out, "Remarkably, considering the large numbers of people who received the SV40-contaminated polio vaccines, no one has conducted a major epidemiological study in the United States to discover whether there is any pattern of illnesses caused by the virus."[148] The little we do know is not good.

When SV40 is given to another species, mice, it can cause sickness. At Johns Hopkins, it was injected in mice who were bred to lack immune systems, and they "developed Kaposi's sarcoma–like tumors, similar to those afflicting many AIDS victims."[149]

As for the simian virus's effect on humans, a number of inconclusive statistical associations have been found.... Research done in Australia in 1968 found a correlation between those who received polio vaccinations and cancers in children past one year of age. Some years later, "German scientists found evidence of SV40 in 30 out of 110 brain tumors [examined], and later reports indicated a jump in the frequency of brain tumors among those [people] who had received vaccine contaminated with SV40."[150]

In conclusion we can say there are two ways that vaccine additives can lead to sickness. The chosen additives may be allergens or disease instigators or the unchosen contaminants may induce states of illness. In a sense these are secondary problems, since additives can be changed and contaminants expunged. What can't be fundamentally altered are the pathogens included in the vaccines that are meant to stimulate antibody production. Now we need to see whether these have any drawbacks.

ADVERSE REACTIONS TO VACCINES THEMSELVES

In our discussion of adverse reactions that have been either tightly or loosely linked to the administration of vaccines, it is not our purpose to offer a laundry list, condemning vaccines right and left as if they were practically tools of the devil. Such a method would be neither true nor illuminating. Not every single vaccine has proven problematic nor would the reader have much patience with an interminable discussion of all those vaccines that have been tied to deteriorating health. What would seem to make more sense would be, that, after noting the suspicious rise in learning disabilities, allergies, and other health impairments after the introduction of childhood inoculations, we shine a light on a couple of vaccines, namely, those that have been employed against whooping cough and hepatitis B, which have very poor showings in terms of the harmful reactions they sometimes produce. Bear in mind, we are highlighting these in particular, but these are not the only vaccines we might have chosen as bad examples.

RISE IN CHRONIC HEALTH PROBLEMS IN CHILDREN

The 21st Report of the United States Department of Education, which covers the school periods 1997–98 to 1998–99 notes an accelerating increase in autism, which has gone up 26 percent in the period, for school-attending children and young adults between six to twenty-one.[151]

This statistic itself may not be accurate. It may be, for example, that the increase is due to a greater percentage of schools reporting or classifying problem youngsters under this heading, rather than a true enlargement of the class. Moreover, there seems no special reason to connect this tragic development to vaccines. What is undeniable, as my next statistics will show further, is that the United States is experiencing an overwhelming blossoming of chronic health disturbances in children.

"The shocking facts that 31 percent of United States children today [1999] suffer from a chronic condition," Dr. Incao testified before the Health Committee of the Ohio House of Representatives, "and that the rate of *disability* in such conditions for children has seen nearly a *fourfold increase* since 1960 ought to seriously challenge our medical research establishment."[152]

Incao was drawing his figures from the health survey conducted yearly since 1957 by the National Center for Health Statistics. The survey also noted that at present 18 percent of children need special healthcare services; while 6.7 percent are seriously disabled by a chronic condition. The most prevalent of these disabling states are respiratory allergies, asthma, and learning disabilities.

More narrowly focusing on autism, Harold Buttram, MD, points to a recent survey conducted by the state of California, which, in the past eleven years, found a 273 percent increase in the condition. He comments further that this tallies with recent studies from other states as well as "reports from the United States Congress on the rapidly increasing needs of classrooms for developmentally delayed children [which] reflect comparable changes across the nation."[153] Dr. Bernard Rimland of the Autism Research Institute sees a statistical overlap between the first uses of MMR vaccine in the United States (in 1975) and in the United Kingdom (in 1988) and a sudden spurt in cases of childhood autism.[154]

The simultaneous appearance of vaccine and a disability is not convincing proof, of course, but since this last specific tie-up, that between MMR and autism, has been more studied than most, let's pause to consider it further.

The study in *Lancet* by Wakefield that we mentioned earlier draws attention to a particular subset of vaccine users. He looked at nursing mothers who were revaccinated with MMR (measles, mumps, rubella vaccine), because rubella protection offered by the original vaccination had worn off or didn't take. He found that these mothers seemed to have a higher than average number of children beset with autistic enterocolitis syndrome, a condition in which autism is paired with bowel disorder. Wakefield feels the intestinal disease is caused by the measles virus included in the MMR. (We will discuss possible causes of autism below). In trying to explain how the measles' component, which is given in a disabled form, can have such a dreadful impact on the child, Wakefield argues that it is not vaccines per se that are to blame, but the unwarranted coupling of more than one weakened pathogen per shot, so that one virus interrupts immune system action against another. He writes,

> The ability of mumps virus to interfere with the cellular immune response to certain strains of measles virus and thereby, in particular combinations, reduce viral clearance [that is, the elimination of the virus by the immune system] and increase the risk of persistent (intestinal) infection, is an intriguing hypothesis [which merits consideration].[155]

Wakefield's work centers on explaining the generation of the bowel disorders in this disease, not the autism. However, the findings of another researcher who looked at MMR vaccine, Dr. Vijendra Singh from the Utah State University Biology Department, may have a bearing on this issue. His tests of autistic children "found that a large majority…had antibodies to brain tissue in the form of antibodies to myelin basic protein."[156]

Myelin is the outer coating of the neurons. A shredding of myelin has been implicated in many brain disorders. So far, what Singh's research implies is that autism can be associated with an auto-immune reaction in which the immune system is attacking its own brain tissues. But here's the frightening finding. Singh noted that "there was a strong correlation between myelin basic protein antibodies and antibodies to measles."[157] In other words, he was finding parallel productions of these two types of antibodies. If there were many myelin antibodies, there were many measles antibodies. The measles antibodies must have been produced in relation to the measles-mumps-rubella vaccine, since none of the children studied had had the measles disease, but almost all had been given the MMR vaccination.

Singh goes no further than noting this disturbing correlation, but Buttram has drawn out the possible causal mechanism that may run from vaccination to a child's collapse into autism. He outlines a possible scenario, beginning with the fact that "protein sequences in the measles virus have been found to have similarities to those found in brain tissues"; which leads him to speculate, "by the process of 'mimicry,' the formation of antibodies against one may cross react with the other."[158]

Such a cross reaction whereby antibodies called out against measles also turned against the body's brain proteins is not as implausible as it might sound. We have shown in *AIDS: A Second Opinion* that human antibodies are not so finely tuned that they will only fasten on one single intruder. They tend to react promiscuously to cells or viruses with similar outer markers.

Furthermore, children have relatively untutored immune systems that become more refined as they mature. Of course, the cross reaction we are imagining here, if it did occur, would also take place if the child had measles. Nevertheless, what is at issue is whether this is occurring with the weakened measles pathogen included in the vaccine. This is an alarming possibility.

Another area of concern for those who think there could be connections between the introduction of national immunization and the overall decline in children's health is the growth in allergies, including asthma, which is often due to allergy. Studies show that in the Western industrial nations, one out of three children has allergies, and as for childhood asthma, some areas have seen a tripling of the numbers affected in the last twenty years. In the United States, the deaths from asthma increased by nearly half (46 percent) in the period running from 1977 to 1991.

"It has not gone unnoticed that the increasing incidence of atopic [allergy-related] disorders has coincided in a time-related fashion with the childhood vaccine programs," writes Buttram. He cites four recent scientific studies that have found "significantly more" allergic disorders among vaccinated children than among those who have had "limited or no vaccines."[159]

In particular, one suspect vaccine here is pertussis, used to immunize against whooping cough. ("Pertussis" is the medical designation for "whooping cough.") Buttram cites four animal and one human experiment that have found increased sensitivity to substances in those who have taken the pertussis inoculation. Allergy, as we know, occurs when the immune system overreacts when exposed to a relatively benign substance, such as a pollen or foodstuff. In one reported experiment, that of Kosceka et al., rats were given egg white alone or with pertussis vaccine. In both cases, the intestines, secretory responses (such as those in the mouth) and other indexes showed an allergic response to further ingestion of the eggs. However, in those rats who had only the food, the response disappeared after two weeks, while those who took the eggs in combination with the vaccine showed the sensitivity for eight months.

How is it that the a pertussis or other vaccinations might make one more susceptible to allergies?

> There is a school of thought that the so-called minor childhood illnesses of former times, including measles, mumps, rubella (German measles), and chicken pox, which entered the body through the mucous membranes, served a necessary and positive purpose in challenging and strengthening the immune system of these membranes.

In contrast, the respective vaccines of these diseases are injected by needle directly into the system of the child, thereby bypassing the mucosal immune system. As a result, mucosal immunity remains relatively weak and stunted in many children, complications of which may be the rapid increase in asthma, eczema, nasal allergies, food allergies and a general pattern of sickness in today's children.[160]

In other words, in the view of thinkers that hold this position, vaccines provide a truncated stimulation of the immune system that leaves it less ready to deal with new infections, allergens, and so on, than it would be if it were beset by the diseases as they occur naturally.

We will have more to say on this topic below when we discuss the different parts of the immune system. We will also look further at pertussis vaccine, which has not only been suggestively linked to allergies but to brain damage and other disabling conditions.

Let us conclude this section by repeating the same complaint noted previously, this time as it comes from the mouth of Philip Incao: "Far from taking a proactive approach toward these disturbing facts," the coincident rise of allergies, learning disabilities, and other conditions among children at the same time as these children were being introduced to multiple inoculations, "our medical establishment remains curiously uninterested in children's *chronic* diseases and instead continues to pursue its narrow focus of using vaccines to eradicate every possible *acute* childhood disease."[161] He might have added, including acute diseases, such as polio, that have more or less disappeared in the West.

And he might have said further, if I may digress a moment, the medical establishment exaggerated interest in vaccines in comparison to other health-enhancing strategies is not surprising from a business point of view. How many drugs are there that a huge population is legally mandated to take? How would it be if every time your son or daughter had a headache, you had to give the child an aspirin or see the child taken away by the state under charge that you were displaying parental neglect? I know that sounds ridiculous. But that is what has sometimes happened to those who refuse to have their children immunized. And since few are either informed enough or brave enough even when informed to go that route, the vaccine makers have little problem with children not getting their shots. Thus as long as children are being born, the pharmaceutical makers have a captive market for their productions. Moreover, given the willingness of our government to mandate new injections, the drug companies have the assurance that some of their new vaccines will also become beneficiaries of this market. Is it any wonder that money for research is poured into this field, while research into say, autism, garners measly funds? Only in vaccines are the successful products guaranteed legal aid from the government in making sure a segment of the population uses their commodities.

PERTUSSIS VACCINE

We have seen there is some evidence that pertussis is linked to allergies. In truth, pertussis might be considered the most unsafe of all the vaccines currently in use. If we look at figures from VAERS—remember this is the organization doctors and other medical personnel are to notify about adverse reactions to vaccines—we find that as of 1998 there were eleven thousand side effects from vaccinations reported per year, including somewhere above 110 deaths. "The majority of deaths are attributed to the pertussis (whooping cough) vaccine."[162] Since only about ten people a year die from whooping cough disease, while about one hundred die from the whooping cough vaccine, we can say the vaccine is out-killing the disease by a ratio of ten to one.

Looking at less violent reactions, we might go back to the testimony of the former Assistant Secretary of Health, Dr. Edward Brandt, who in 1985 said about pertussis vaccine, "Every year 35,000 children suffer neurological reactions because of this vaccine."[163] Typical reactions are convulsions or high-pitched screaming. Dr. Keith Block, after analyzing a study in *Pediatrics* journal, says these neurological reactions are experienced by one in 175 children who get the vaccination.[164]

There is little chance, by the way that figures of deaths and adverse reactions to vaccines, such as those we culled from VAERS, are over-reported. Just the opposite. Good evidence has it that under-reporting is the norm. The FDA has calculated that only about 10 percent of adverse reactions to vaccines that occur are brought to the attention of health agencies. This calculation has been vouched for by two studies from the National Vaccine Information Center. The Center also conducted an in-depth look at notifications of adverse reactions given by New York City doctors. It found that only one in forty physicians bothered to report them, even when deaths resulted.[165]

While the physical problems that can result from getting a shot of pertussis vaccine are not in doubt, the vaccine's utility against whooping cough is. A study by B. Trollfors, a Swedish epidemiologist, concluded, "No difference [in whooping cough disease-induced fatalities] can be discerned when countries with high, low, and zero immunization rates were compared."[166] Trollfors's analysis of three Western nations (West Germany, England, and Wales) showed further that deaths from the disease were higher when these countries had high immunization rates than when immunization of the population was less thorough.

Let's go back to a topic brought up about pertussis vaccine in earlier discussion. We mentioned before that the DPT inoculation had been associated by some researchers with SIDS, sudden infant death syndrome. To be more precise at this point, it is the pertussis vaccine included in the DPT package, which has been seen as behind the upsurge in mortality from SIDS. Deaths from this syndrome are estimated to be between five thousand to ten thousand a year in the United States. My earlier comment was that there was no hard and fast evidence on this vaccine/SIDS association. Still the following two concurrences should give pause: First, a study of United States children found that the highest incidence of SIDS occurred when the infant was either two or four months old. It is at these two ages that the DPT injections are given. Second, "in the mid-seventies Japan raised their [sic] vaccination age from two months to two years; their incidence of SIDS dropped dramatically.[167]

Aside from direct evidence (vaccine-related deaths noted by VAERS) and correlation (such as the two relationships just mentioned), there is also indirect evidence of a tie between the pertussis vaccine and impairment. Buttram finds it both interesting and disturbing that when animal experiments are being carried out in which it is necessary to induce encephalitis in the subjects, such as that of Munoz et al. on mice, then to create this type of brain damage, the animals are given a derivative of pertussis vaccine![168] This certainly doesn't speak well for the safety of the preparation.

While evidence seems to be piling up suggesting that pertussis may have troubling effects on the health of children, there is also evidence that this whole situation could have been avoided if the vaccine had been more thoroughly vetted. Writing in *Adverse Drug Reactions & Toxicology Review*, Wakefield and Montgomery underline that the drug trials which preceded approval of DPT vaccine for use kept check on the health of the inoculated subjects of the trials for a maximum of twenty-eight days, and often for less time. In the article, Wakefield and Montgomery emphasized that "such short periods of observation were totally inadequate to detect delayed reactions, including pervasive developmental decay (autism), immune deficiencies, and inflammatory bowel disease."[169]

If we were to make up wanted posters featuring the vaccines to which can be attributed the most danger, that is ones whose occasionally calamitous health effects are generally recognized, even by the industry, then pertussis vaccine would be Public Enemy Number One. While showing itself weak against the disease it is supposed to be protecting us from, it has been associated with autism, allergies, SIDS, and other health imbalances. However, aside from recorded adverse reactions, the studies that suggest a link between pertussis vaccine and health impairments are speculative. Opposed studies have argued against many of these associations. Still, the circumstantial evidence seems strong enough, if it is added to the high level of acknowledged impairments from the vaccine received by VAERS, to make this vaccine seem both unreliable and unnecessary. This is something that can be said for few other vaccines, although among that few would be the one for hepatitis B.

HEPATITIS B VACCINE

A moment ago, we mentioned that if a new vaccine is approved by the FDA, it represents a gold mine for the lucky maker. We should qualify that by adding that this would be contingent on state governments getting with the program and mandating all school children get inoculated with the new offering. Moreover, this itself would depend on making the disease that the vaccine is providing protection against seem a scourge, whether it had previously seemed to belong to this category or not.

We can see these processes at work with the hepatitis B vaccine, which was introduced in 1990, and is now required by thirty-six states as a condition of school attendance. This vaccine was mandated in the face of some skepticism. After all, it is a disease usually confined to certain high-risk groups, and is anything but prevalent. In 1996, for example, there were only 279 cases of the disease in people below the age of fourteen. In 90 percent of these cases, as well as in the some 10,350 cases suffered by older people that year, the sufferer experienced a mild flu-like disease and threw off the illness through the efforts of his or her immune system.

Those who came down with the illness generally fit into the following high-risk categories, as identified by the CDC: drug addicts, those (straight or gay) who have multiple sexual partners, children of immigrants from certain areas, healthcare workers, and newborns whose mothers are infected. Offhand, it would seem money and work could be saved if only those belonging to these groups were vaccinated. After all, as we have already shown, the WHO's great campaign to eradicate smallpox around the globe depended on just such a strategy of identifying and inoculating those who were at particular risk, in this case because they had contact with a disease sufferer. Broad-gauge immunization was found to be not as effective as selective targeting of those who needed the vaccine.

However, in dealing with hepatitis B, the CDC thinks broad gauge is better. Conservative researcher Tom Bethel, quoting the agency's reasoning behind its endorsement of universal childhood vaccination, states, "The CDC explains that it has 'generally not been feasible' to identify people "engaged in high-risk behaviors." Instead, the agency recommended "making hepatitis B vaccine a part of routine vaccination schedules for infants."[170]

Bethel reacts to this CDC position with the acerbic (if easily misinterpreted) fulmination, "In other words, the risk of adverse events must be borne by innocent infants, who can be singled out on maternity wards, because the sex and drug addicts can't be expected to identify themselves."[171] Such a statement has to be understood literally. Bethel is not saying, for instance, that the sexually promiscuous won't identify themselves and be vaccinated. This is a separate matter. Nor is he arguing that every high-risk person fits in these groups of "addicts." Nurses and others would also be high-risk, but they could easily be identified and vaccinated. All he is saying is that the CDC is basing its policy on this interpretation of certain groups' probable behavior.

Unfortunately, Bethel's plaintive complaint offers more heat than light. It may seem ethically wrong to make the fate of children depend on the behavior of addicts, but the significant questions should be not on what the CDC says (Bethel's focus), but on whether what it say is accurate. In this situation, the relevant queries would be, granted these addicts won't self-identify—and that is a supposition, not an objective finding—then, (1) Is it likely they will pass the infection on to children, and (2) if they will, is massive immunization the best way to stop them from so doing?

From what we have already said, it can be seen that our answers to these questions would support neither of the underlying rationalizations for inoculating infants. (1) Judging by the low level of the hepatitis B–infected who are fourteen or younger in comparison to the great number of infected adults and young adults, there is minimal transmission of the disease from the old to the young. (2) As the WHO smallpox campaign illustrates, even if older people were passing the disease to children at a much greater rate than they are, massive vaccinations would not be the best way to get at the problem. Selective immunization has proven itself the better method of disease control.

Now, to continue with what was mentioned a moment ago, to get a new vaccine approved, it is not sufficient to have the CDC provide flimsy justifications. There needs to be the inspiration of public fear. Making people think that they are putting their children's health at risk if they don't get them inoculated and, more importantly, if they don't see to it that everyone else's children are inoculated, is what makes them willing to approve the further intrusion of the government into their lives.

We can pick up again the writing of Hyde and Forsyth to see how, when it comes to creating fear, vaccine promoters fall to the task with a will. In their discussion of hepatitis B, they begin by telling over a litany of death and disease, mentioning an estimated four thousand to five thousand deaths a year, and an estimated one hundred thousand new infections. However, although they are firm believers in infant vaccinations, nowhere is there a mention of how many of these hepatitis B patients are youngsters. Thus, the fact that it turns out very few children get the disease is left in the shadows.

The exposition continues with an anxiety-producing list of all the ways the infection can be spread. We learn, "sharing toothbrushes, razors, and washcloths can also transmit hepatitis B," for example, and it can be picked up from "contaminated beaches and in shellfish."[172] All of this is true, but it leaves out of sight the facts that very few children get the infection and, typically, those that do get it have impaired immune systems. The authors then tell the story of a girl, Arkesha Johnson of Minneapolis, who never got the hepatitis shot. When she felt stomach pains, her mother took her to a health center. "After some tests, the girl was taken to the hospital. She never went home again," having died from hepatitis B infection.[173] This is a tragic story, but when such narratives are inserted in examinations of particular diseases, as this one is in the discussion of hepatitis B, the presumption is that they are representative, that is, many cases more or less like the one narrated could be told.

Our contention is that the following story is more representative than was Johnson's. Lyla Rose Belkin was a lively, healthy, engaged five-month-old baby. One night, though, she seemed agitated. She fell asleep and never woke up. An autopsy could find no illness aside from cranial swelling, and her death was labeled as due to SIDS. "A few hours before Lyla's death, she had been inoculated with the hepatitis B vaccine."[174]

This is one case of many where adverse physical reactions followed immediately on reception of the vaccine. "Since July 1990, 17,497 cases of hospitalizations, injuries and deaths in America following hepatitis B vaccination have been reported to VAERS," and in this group fall 146 deaths, half of whom (73) are of children.[175] Remember, too, infant Lyla's death would not find its way into these statistics since the doctor in charge stated she died of SIDS (a medical convenience for unexplainable deaths). This doctor refused to entertain the possibility the vaccine could have played a part in the little girl's collapse.

In published reports, notice has been given of forty-five different adverse reactions to hepatitis B vaccine, including, occlusion of the central retinal nerve, cerebral hemorrhage, pulmonary bleeding, bleeding diarrhea, visual loss, and rheumatoid arthritis. The vaccine has also been connected to various auto-immune/neurological disorders such as Guillain-Barre syndrome, autism, and central nervous system demylinization, the last being the problem we also so associated with measles vaccine.[176]

Some of these conditions manifested shortly after administration of the vaccine, while others took weeks to appear. As with the suspicious MMR vaccine, trials of hepatitis B vaccine "monitored children only for four or five days after vaccination," thus never confronting the possibility that effects might have appeared after some time lapse following the reception of the vaccine.[177]

While to the public, the CDC responded to gadflies' questioning of the safety of this vaccine by issuing a clean bill of health, misgivings have surfaced within the agency. "A leaked internal CDC memo...[states] a meeting at the agency in 1997 discussed 'possible association' between the vaccine and MS [multiple sclerosis] and recommended a 'case-control study' of the association."[178]

We can see that even within the medical establishment there are people who look askance at the safety of this vaccine. You've probably heard the expression in which someone said a particular experience "made a believer" out of him or her. Well, her experience with hepatitis B vaccine "made a doubter" out of Dr. Bonnie Dunbar.

A few years ago, a professor at the Baylor College of Medicine in Houston was honored by the NIH for her work on vaccines. Then her brother was given a hepatitis B inoculation. Shortly thereafter he experienced MS-like symptoms. As she testified, "His problems have been attributed to the hepatitis B vaccine by over a dozen different specialists of unquestionable medical expertise."[179] He is permanently and totally impaired. At this point, she began to speak out against the overuse and misuse of vaccinations, for example, testifying at the Texas Public Health Board. At that meeting, she prefaced her remarks on the hazards of vaccine, with the following cutting comment, " I am sure that some of my colleagues would not approve of my appearance. Especially those that are benefiting handsomely from pharmaceutical company income as consultants and expert witnesses while carrying on vaccine clinical trials."[180] She is emphasizing that not only vaccine producers but scientists who work in the field of immunization stand to gain when new vaccines are approved.

More and more people are joining Dunbar in doubting the value of hepatitis B and some of the less savory vaccines we have discussed in these pages, not only because they are known to or expected of causing so many adverse reactions, but because of the dawning understanding of how they may possibly unbalance the immunity system and intrude into genetic material.

VACCINE INTERFERENCE WITH CELLULAR DNA

One danger arising from vaccine use is rooted in the fact, already highlighted, that viruses and bacteria move around genetic material laterally, shifting bits between themselves and also into their hosts' DNA. Of course, of the two parasites, it is the virus that would more likely be monkeying with human genetic code since its method of action is to invade a host cell and then set its own DNA to work, incorporating it in the DNA in the host's nucleus.

So, let's keep the focus on viruses. Those included in vaccines are weakened so that they will not cause a full-blown illness, but weakening does not mean they have lost the ability to swap genes. "Thus there is the potential that disease viruses will incorporate their own…genetic material into the chromosomes of the children that have been vaccinated."[181] Little research has been done on whether this could be taking place. Further, as Buttram stresses, even if scientists wanted to investigate this topic, it is debatable whether they have the technology to identify viral contamination of cellular DNA.

A few disquieting experiments have probed this area. One done in Italy on patients who had post-vaccination central nervous system diseases compared them with control groups. Of those with the diseases, 73.3 percent were found to have genetic damage.[182] Veterans suffering from the Gulf War syndrome have also been studied for genetic problems. A three-year research project done at the University of Michigan discovered that of twenty-four military personnel affected by this syndrome, "50 percent were found to have abnormal RNA indicating chromosomal damage."[183]

In neither case, is it possible to say what role, if any , vaccines played in provoking the genetic damage. Indeed, the Michigan study presupposes toxic chemicals are largely responsible for the RNA alterations. Currently, the whole area is hazy.

However, as Dr. Joshua Lederberg, leading expert on new diseases, notes, this haze may contain deadly shoals. He writes, "In point of fact, we [are practicing] biological engineering on a rather large scale by use of live vaccines in mass immunization campaigns." He bids us bear in mind that vaccine making is still not very sophisticated. "Crude virus preparations, such as some in common use at present time, are also vulnerable to frightful mishaps of contamination and misidentification."[184]

His statement is not meant to connote that if vaccines were made in a less chancy, more competent manner, they would then be hazard free. Even the most fastidiously produced vaccine, if it relies on live virus, still threatens with the possibility of gene transfer from virus to host. If such a state of affairs does come to be and viral genetic material is joined with human DNA or RNA, two health problems can be envisioned. The appearance of alien matter in the gene could prompt antibody countermeasures or, if antibodies ignore this material, it could remain as a "time bomb," apt to cause disabilities farther down the road.

Walene James presents an illuminating synopsis of how the first possibility would be played out. Once a live virus—and most antiviral vaccines use live but weakened viruses—gets into a cell, it attaches its

> own genetic material as an extra particle or "episome" to the genome (half set of chromosomes and their genes) of the host cell and [begins] replicating along with it. This allows the host cell to continue its own normal functions for the most part but imposes on it additional instructions for the synthesis of viral proteins. "The persistence of live viruses or other foreign antigens within the cells of the host therefore cannot fail to provoke auto-immune phenomena, because destroying the infected cells is now the only possible way that this constant antigenic challenge can be removed from the body."[185]

To explain further, immune system components do not have the facility of actually going into cells and snooping around for viruses, but they can detect the presence of unlawful (non-self) material inside the cell by screening from outside. If they sense such matter has invaded a cell, they quickly dispatch the aptly named killer cells to destroy the whole configuration, cell and invaders dying together.

Such killing in itself is no cause for alarm. When someone gets a viral disease, such as a cold, this type of cell elimination takes place as part of our natural defense mechanism. Yet, there is a difference between antibody reaction to a normally invasive virus and one that has wrapped itself into cellular genetic machinery. When detector antibodies discover, say, cells infected with influenza virus, what has alerted them to the untoward situation is the presence of viral replicants in the cell's fluid. The first-invading virus has made numerous copies of itself, preparatory to exploding the cell (as so many of the viruses overtax the cell's holding capacity) and flooding back into the bloodstream. However, where the viral material is not making more viruses but simply sitting in the cell's DNA, it is possible, some scientists theorize, that the detector antibodies may get befuddled. The detector recognizes a foreign element in the cell, but this element is tied into a self element. In certain cases, this illicit combination will disturb the perceptual abilities of the detector. It will send out killer cells against even innocent cells because of this confusion. The end result is an auto-immune disease in which the immune system goes haywire destroying uncontaminated cells. An article in *Science* describes the situation in these words, "The DNA vaccine gene may incorporate into and damage human chromosomes and the vaccines may prompt the body to make anti-DNA antibodies, which are found in people with auto-immune disorders such as lupus."[186]

And there is yet another problem imbricated here. Think for a moment of the disease shingles, which causes painful, scabby rash. No one can get shingles, a disease of older people, unless they have first had chickenpox. The chickenpox virus, once it has caused the original disease and been vanquished by a person's immunity, leaves remnants in the nervous system. Later in life, when a person is under stress or has other problems that lead to weakened health, the virus blooms in a new form, producing shingles. This whole pathology indicates that viruses can take up positions in our bodies where they bide their time, awaiting a deficient internal state before they make a new manifestation. If a virus manages to incorporate into cell DNA without getting the attention of the immune system, it may be that, years later, in some way not yet understood, it will begin either signaling the immune system that there is something wrong (causing an autoimmune disease) or create some malfunction in the genetic wiring (issuing in a disease such as cancer). It this possibility of viral genes derived from vaccines hiding in our DNA and later erupting in somatic disease that caused Dr. Robert Mendelsohn to ask, "Have we traded mumps and measles [which vaccines now protect us from] for cancer and leukemia?"[187]

The danger that viral DNA will become entangled with our own chromosomes, which is so far only speculation, is based on two evident facts. The first is that we know viruses can hook up with our DNA under certain circumstances. It is certainly well established that they are adept at shifting segments of genetic material around. The second is that we are now plagued by a slew of illnesses, from cancer to MS to ALS, which cause death and horrifying disabilities, involve some disturbance of our own cellular mechanism, and are of unknown cause.

Perhaps, if these speculations are correct, further thought and research will provide a more concrete idea of how such disease processes work. In any case, more is known about our next topic, how vaccine use may end up unbalancing the immune system.

DISTORTION OF THE IMMUNE SYSTEM BY VACCINES

At the beginning of our discussion of immunizations, we alluded to the possibility that when given to infants or children, it may be that vaccines don't stimulate the immune system as fully as would a mild attack of disease. Later, when commenting on allergies, we presented the situation more specifically by drawing attention to the body's different reactions to airborne disease, depending on whether it appeared naturally or through a vaccine. When a child comes down with such a disease, one like measles, the immune components that stand guard in the mucosal lining of the nose, mouth, lungs, and intervening parts of the respiratory system will get full play as they mobilize against the intrusive pathogens. Obviously, if the child gets an attenuated vaccine version of the germ injected into the blood by a needle, the nose and lungs will be left out of the loop, as it were. Though the inoculated child has had the disease, as far as the respiratory mechanism is concerned, it never happened. The immune responses of this part of the body have not been given any practice coping with intruders.

This is bad enough but there is a another difficulty, which touches upon the very foundation of immunity. Philip Incao has written an articulate discussion of this issue in a piece titled "How Vaccination Works," and I will draw extensively on it here.

Current research sees the immune system to be made up of two complementary parts. The humoral segment (more technically, the Th2 function) is what we previously called the detector. Its antibodies work their way through the body examining the markings on cells to make sure they are identifiably indigenous. If they are not, the other segment of the immune system, cell-mediated immunity (Th1), takes over, destroying, surrounding (and thus decommissioning) or ejecting foreign elements. It is this "inflammatory" response that is felt by the affected individual as symptoms such as fever, pain, rashes, diarrhea, runny nose, and so on.

These two components of immunity function well in tandem, one monitoring for invaders, the other running any off that are located. Think about this. What would be the outcome if one of these components stopped functioning? Although this doesn't happen when vaccinations are given, the effect of a vaccination is to temporarily blot out the activity of part of our natural immunity.

> A vaccination consists of introducing a disease agent or disease antigen into an individual's body *without* causing the disease. If the disease agent provoked the *whole* immune system into action it *would* cause all the symptoms of the disease!... So the trick of a vaccination is to stimulate the immune system just enough so that it makes antibodies and "remembers" the disease antigen but not so much that it provokes an acute inflammatory response by the cellular immune system and make us sick with the disease we're trying to prevent. Thus a vaccination works by stimulating *very much* the antibody production (Th2) and by stimulating *very little* or not at all the digesting and discharging function of the cellular immune system (Th1).[188]

This would be the effect at whatever age the vaccination is given. However, in the view of vaccine critics, giving a child a string of inoculations and thus constantly exercising only one part of its immunity, is courting disaster. Buttram explains that both the Th1 and Th2 immunity systems are governed by Th lymphocytes, types of white blood cells. "Early in life these 'naïve' or uncommitted Th lymphocytes are differentiated into either armed Th1 cells...or armed Th2 cells.... This initial differentiation...has a critical impact on the outcome of adaptive immune response."[189] Once a particular bias of the system is locked in, shown by the assignment of lymphocytes to either branch of the immune system in childhood, it is difficult or impossible to shift the balance later.

Moreover, as a child matures, if he or she has been breastfed, there is a natural transition from antibodies loaned from the mother through her milk to those that, as the child is weaned, are created by the girl or boy as diseases are contracted and overcome. The arbitrary injection with vaccines during nursing ignores this natural sequence and transects the shift from (mother-supplied) passive to active immunity for the child.[190]

Let's revert to a point already noted, which is that the insertion of the virus or other pathogen directly into the bloodstream allows it to bypass its normal entry point. (We are leaving out of consideration, of course, the diseases that do start out in the blood, such as those injected by mosquitoes.) We can follow James in noting that this turns the normal immune response sequence on its head. By using a needle to get the germ in the body, vaccinators "accomplish what the entire immune system seems to have evolved to prevent."[191] Mouth, throat, nose, lungs, stomach, intestines, all these organs are filled with first-line defenses to capture and expunge illicit entities. If an intruder slips past these defenses (assuming they are in good working order), we can say that it is particularly hardy, wily, or possessive of some other superior ability. To put this in other terms, the blood-borne immune system has been developed as a second-line defense to chase down a selective batch of extra-capable parasites. By getting viruses, such as measles, into the blood without making them prove their worth in reaching that point, the immune factors in the blood are faced with relatively innocuous invaders. Although there is no research on this, one can wonder along with James: What will be the effect of consistently priming blood-borne immune responses with germs that are some degrees less deadly than those that will be met with in the real world?

At this point, we need to distinguish between differing viewpoints on the correct balance of immune system elements. We saw that for Incao, the hazard of weighting the immune function in favor of antibody production is that the system will lose its equipoise. Buttram counters that it is better if the immune system is slightly prejudiced toward one component of the system, with pride of place being given to cellular immunity. He writes, "In both the *New England Journal of Medicine* and *Thorax*, articles have appeared stating that a healthy immune system has a 'bias' toward the Th1 system."[192] As we have seen, it is just this Th1 system that the stimulation provided by vaccines downplays.

Although these writers disagree on exactly what balance should be achieved in a properly modulated immune system, they are as one in seeing that vaccination is creating an immune organization that responds to the artificial way it receives pathogens by overcompensating on the Th2 side. As Incao pithily remarks, far from boosting the immune system in toto, "What in reality is prevented [by vaccination] is not the disease but the ability of our cellular immune system to *manifest, to respond to* and *to overcome* the disease!"[193] Although one may find him a little harsh in this passage, since in most cases, at least short term, the disease is prevented by immunization, even as (possibly) overall immunity is warped, one can hardly object to the sentence with which he follows this comment. It runs, "There is no system of the human being, from mind to muscles to immune system, which gets stronger through avoiding challenges, but only through *overcoming* challenges."[194]

Here, also, a great deal of groundwork needs to be done to actually prove all these assertions. Studies plotting numbers of cells from each component of the immune system in both vaccinated and unvaccinated children would be of major importance in this respect. However, it would seem there is little doubt that this type of immune system distortion is likely to arise, given that vaccine is premised on just such a partial activation.

An advocate of childhood immunization would see the fact that a child avoids the more hurtful incursions of a disease through inoculation as a plus. As we've seen, this is shortsighted.

We can use the concepts presented by noted child psychologist Bruno Bettelheim in his book *The Uses of Enchantment* for the purpose of an analogy. Bettelheim argues that the classic European fairy tales presented children with rather grim and horrifying images. A wolf would eat a grandmother, a witch would fatten up a child for a cannibalistic meal, a dead mother would be replaced with an unsympathetic stepmother. In Bettelheim's view, it is the very roughness of these stories that gives them major value as educators. They acquaint children with the harsh facts of life that sooner or later would have to be faced. Rather than letting children remain innocent until they have their illusions shattered in adolescence, the fairy tales give even the youngest child a fair knowledge of the whole of life, both its moments of glory and times of misery.

Coupled with Bettelheim's literary reflection are some rather unflattering words he has to say about the place of fairy tales in modern American culture. Rather than leaving these narratives in their pristine state, with all their unpleasant features intact, American purveyors of children's tales, from Walt Disney to the TV networks, have pulled the sting from the ancient stories, sanitizing and removing their upsetting elements. But, dispelling all the gloom, they have also taken away the most beneficial lessons from the tales, and at the same time, they have helped children gain a more realistic view of themselves. Bettelheim puts it like this:

> There is a widespread refusal to let children know the source of much that goes wrong in life is due to our very own natures—the propensity of all men for acting aggressively, asocially, [and so on].... Instead, we want our children to believe that all men are inherently good. But children know that *they* are not always good.... This contradicts what they are told by their parents, and therefore makes the child a monster in his own eyes.[195]

By giving more realistic versions of human nature and life experiences, fairy tales had historically served as a psychic toughener for children.

The parallel to the practice of immunization is not far to seek. Just as fairy tales were useful in preparing children for the real world by giving them some acquaintance with its crueler aspects, so childhood diseases used to give the child's immune system a vigorous workout, preparing it for the more violent stresses it would probably face later in life. But now American society has found ways to preempt both these learning routes, providing instead milquetoast children's literature and the equivalent unstressful way to encounter disease. It has been argued that this leaves the child doubly unprepared, unforearmed before the psychic and pathogenic buffeting to come.

Moreover, paradoxically, in order to make sure the public agrees to and walks in step with these systems of programmed innocence, there has been a resort to subterfuge and coercion. For vaccines, as we will see, coercion has appeared in such instances as when children are barred from attending school unless they are vaccinated, just as in the 1960s Disneyland had security guards, acting on orders from the top, who made sure hippies and others who did not look sufficiently well-groomed were not allowed entrance to the park, where harmony *must* reign.

SUBTERFUGES IN THE PROMOTION OF VACCINES

It perhaps follows from what we have said about the money to be made from vaccine sales and about how scare campaigns are orchestrated to get states to adopt universal child immunization that vaccine promoters may not always be overly scrupulous in what information they provide about vaccines' characteristics.

In fact in running over how the need for childhood inoculations with hepatitis B vaccine was promoted, we noticed the use of somewhat underhanded methods. A terrible series of events were highlighted, in which a girl, who hadn't been immunized, died from the disease. While the inclusion of such a case, subtly hinted that deaths likes hers were occurring all the time, the very low incidence of childhood hepatitis B infection (shown by national statistics) suggest that a case like the girl's is highly unrepresentative.

Also the material, in making a case for childhood vaccination, presented aggregated statistics (ones that lumped together everyone who got the disease) of deaths from hepatitis B. This would lead you to believe a good percentage of the deaths were of children. This was not the case.

Such minor tampering will occur whenever it is necessary to put facts in the best light, and is, perhaps, excusable. However, one thing you would think would not be fiddled with would be the actual success rates of vaccines. These can be tremendously dramatic as are these from Hyde and Forsyth, "Before the measles vaccine was approved in 1963, more than five hundred thousand cases of measles occurred in the United States each year.... After the vaccine was available, the number of cases dropped to less than two thousand over a period of two decades."[196] Such figures are always trotted out to chart the great strides made in the elimination of disease once vaccines were discovered and employed. Few would doubt these figures. Yet, what we want to touch on now is how in some cases slight discrepancies will be found at either end of these statistics: both in original estimates of how many people are suffering from the condition before the vaccine was in wide use as well as the number who are still getting the disease after mass inoculation has been instituted.

As to why statistics at the front end of the process may not be as unassailable as they seem, we can repeat some interesting findings of Professor Gordon Stewart concerning the early days of the polio vaccination campaign. Here is how Michael Verney-Elliot reports Stewart's findings:

> In the USA during the late forties, there was a noticeable increase in polio cases. This prompted the authorities to pay a bounty of $25 to GPs reporting any suspected case of polio, treating it as a notifiable disease. The numbers of cases of polio shot up, causing a national panic. Any stiff neck or slight limp was reported. Curiously, at the same time, the official number of cases of asceptic meningitis, which shares some symptoms with polio, and previously reached some twenty-five thousand annually nationwide, disappeared completely. A whole disease just vanished.[197]

As can be seen here, diseases often overlap in symptoms, and so it is possible to fudge on diagnosing them. Stewart avers that patients' would be variably classified as affected with either polio or asceptic meningitis, no matter which disease they really had, according to which was more profitable or acceptable in the prevailing climate.

We noted previously that the same sort of thing went on at the back end of case reporting. When Jenner saw that a few vaccinated patients would come down with what looked like smallpox, he relabeled it as "spurious cowpox." In the eyes of researcher Meryl Dorey, this same sort of reclassification of diseases occurred after prevalent vaccination, abetted, curiously enough, by the increased discriminatory power of our diagnostic tools. As he told me,

> At that time [the 1960s], testing for the [smallpox] virus became more sophisticated. You no longer were suffering necessarily from smallpox. They would test it and find it had different DNA. You'd have monkeypox or camelpox or some other form of pox. But it was still called variola, which is smallpox....
>
> Clinically, the disease is exactly the same as smallpox. It has the same progression. It looks exactly the same. If you put a smallpox victim next to a monkeypox victim, you will not be able to tell the difference. As a matter of fact, with this outbreak of monkeypox in Africa [occurring at the time of our conversation]...they are suggesting that they use the smallpox vaccine again. Funny—if it's not the same disease, why would the vaccine be effective?[198]

Dorey's argument is that in order to preserve the unsullied reputation of the smallpox vaccination campaign, scientists have re-categorized patients, making those who would once have been seen as struck down by smallpox as sickened by one sort of animal pox or another.

The same type of thing happened in the *pas de deux* between polio and asceptic meningitis. While, asceptic meningitis trended down at the same time as physicians were being paid for identifying polio cases, once polio was said to have been conquered, it moved in the opposite direction. Stewart recounts, "When the polio epidemic had abated, the credit [for the success] being given to Salk and Sabin's polio vaccines...the numbers of meningitis cases returned to their previous level."[199]

We are not putting these examples of statistical manipulation forward as serious disproof of the value of vaccination. What we are seeing is the way science becomes ideology. As scientists, vaccine promoters should be able to admit that vaccines are neither foolproof nor flawless. But as ideologists—and I believe medical personnel are pulled into this role as soon as health-care conjoins with business and government—they have to hold up impossible ideals of vaccines' harmlessness and effectiveness. These are concepts more at home in public relations offices than in the laboratory. And once such a position is taken, in which vaccines will be defended to the point of ignoring weaknesses in their operation, then it is a short step to stifling those who disbelieve in them.

COERCION AND THE VACCINATION OF CHILDREN

Most people who send their children to be inoculated have not investigated the safety and effectiveness of the procedure. Unless they possess an independent spirit and the free time to dig into the matter—and probably more people possess the former than the latter—they will accept the pro-industry standpoint of the mass media and the government. Besides, they need to have a record showing that their children have gotten their shots so they can start them at school.

This last point is the clincher. State governments mandate vaccinations for children and make outlaws of parents who resist. Just as soldiers have been court-martialed for refusing the anthrax vaccination, so parents who do not want their kids inoculated have been sued for child neglect. They have even been denied medical care if they refuse the needle.

James recounts what happened when a mother took her toddler to see a doctor. When the physician asked if the child was vaccinated, the mother replied she was waiting until the girl had grown older and had a more developed immune system to have them given. "The doctor excused himself to consult with his colleagues in the office. When he came back, he said, 'I'm sorry, but we don't treat children who aren't immunized.'"[200]

A number of states have even passed laws to keep those youngsters who don't go to public schools, such as who are home schooled or attending private schools, from slipping through the net.

We are not about to launch into a lament over government encroachment into our private lives, although that is a topic worth pursuing. What we want to briefly reflect upon is medicine and authoritarianism.

Imagine if you will another way of going about immunizations. Say each school took the parents of its new students aside, explained the pros and cons of vaccination, and told them why the school thinks it is needed. Then the parents made a decision. Whatever they decided, even if every single parent agreed to the vaccinations, there would be a radical change in how healthcare is being provided. Such a procedure would be a way to cultivate a more scientifically engaged citizenry; moreover a group that felt it had an input into and stake in both the educational and public health bureaucracy.

What we have instead is health by fiat. Parents are not gently led to see the values of vaccination (as it appears to public health personnel), but stampeded into compliance. We can wonder whether such a way of doing medicine, even if the procedure being plumped for were unquestionably right, is humanely correct. Take the situation mentioned by James when she is discussing vaccine-damaged children, "In many case...the [female] parent was opposed to, or at least hesitant about, immunizations but let herself be pressured into consenting." For James, the parent's nervousness is communicated to the youngster. "There is a bond between mother and child that is particularly strong during those early years, and any anxiety and resentment the parent feels can be picked up by the child."[201] If the child fears the shot, this may prime it for an adverse reaction.

Some may find this a bit farfetched, feeling that a baby's immune system is unlikely to be affected by a mother's misgivings about a shot. Still, I think few would gainsay our broader position which is that the doctor-patient or nurse-patient relationship enters in some fundamental way into the healing process, and whether this relationship is coercive or democratic will have impact on the ultimate consequences of the medical intervention.

Let's move on to one other point worth making on this subject. Suppose that rather than playing by the rules of immunization, which would have the family quietly and uncomplainingly doing as bidden, it turns out that the parents are informed and would like to open a discourse about the value of vaccines.

This is precisely what happened to Walene James. Her grown daughter did not want to let her child be vaccinated and was taken to court by the state of Virginia. What the grown daughter wanted to do, aided by her mother who was something of an expert on the dangers of immunization, was to fight on principle, bringing experts and documents to court that disputed the value of vaccines. She was told she needed a lawyer, so she consulted one. "He asked Tanya [the daughter] about her financial resources. When he found these were inadequate, he recommended she join the Christian Science Church."[202] Members of this church were exempt from the immunization law because vaccinations conflicted with their religious beliefs. Tanya was being counseled to use this group, not as a philosophical path, but as an escape hatch. (The state attorney who was prosecuting the case, obliquely gave her the same directions as a way of sidestepping a court hearing.)

As we can see, the concern of the legal system is to avoid drawn-out debate. There are good reasons for this, seeing as the courts are clogged with suits and tend to be understaffed. Besides, if a case is to be argued, legal procedures will only run smoothly if they are conducted by trained professionals, namely, lawyers. There are good reasons, then, for damping controversy and restricting most people from participating. Still, the results of such emphases is that we arrive at a system that is streamlined and efficient but shuts out any citizen who has something valuable to contribute.

If this were the only realm of society that erred on the side of timidity, the situation would not be so bad. However, in institution after institution, there seems to be a conspiracy *to* silence those with substantially different perspectives. (It's important to keep in mind that the tendency we are highlighting here is that of avoiding forthright discussion of any charged issue, not just vaccination.)

Walene James narrates this example of "academic freedom." She notes, "A friend of mine was teaching a course in early childhood development at Cuyahoga College in Ohio," which was designed for parents with kids in Head Start. The friend got to the topic of Ohio's vaccination laws, which exempt children for such reasons as ill health and the parents' religious beliefs. Soon after, James continues, "My friend was called into the [instructional] supervisor's office and told that the policy of the college was that vaccinations were mandatory and not to tell students otherwise!"[203]

In this instance, an administrator is objecting to a teacher simply informing parents of their rights. Imagine if the instructor had tried to talk about the drawbacks of immunization.

Another situation, one with much broader implications, exposes the same type of delimitation of all-sided discussion as it occurs in politics. In 1993, the Senate debated a bill that would institute greater surveillance of families to insure as few as possible avoided vaccination of their children. It passed unanimously. Since the legislators are not experts on medical issues, they needed to consult those from the field to get a sense of the value of vaccinations.

> House and Senate hearings on the above legislation barred healthcare professionals concerned about the safety and efficacy of vaccinations from testifying. Parents [whose children had been damaged through immunization]

were purposely forbidden to speak....Who was permitted to testify? Four presidents of companies that produce vaccines, the [pro-vaccine] American Academy of Pediatrics and [pro-vaccine] public health officials.... At least one TV network news channel I saw [James says] made much of the "fact" that vested interests such as the AMA weren't permitted to testify at the meetings.[204]

Our two examples can't substitute for sociological research, but they do at least suggest that there are forces in these varied institutions arrayed against the airing of a broad range of views. An increase of democracy, as would be symbolized here by opening classrooms and legislative hearings to oppositional perspectives, would tend to produce sloppy and conflictual goings-on, the kind large organizations find abhorrent.

Just as the older scientific paradigm is atomized, hierarchical, and one-dimensional, so are the social networks that support its practice. In contrast, the new paradigm emphasizes emergent properties (whereby higher levels of organization have qualities not derivable from their components) and interconnectedness. Medical organizations that are tied to the development of this paradigm (ideally) should interject into healthcare more choice, informed decision making, and constructive dissension. We will say more about this in the book's conclusion, but, while we're minded to make recommendations, let's make a few more as a way to sum up our position on vaccines.

NECESSARY CHANGES

■ We should first put a hold on the use of the more disastrous vaccines, "disastrous" in terms of high number of adverse effects recorded with their use.

These would include the experimental anthrax vaccines used on military personnel. We also have to rethink the use of vaccines for illnesses that are not occurring in the United States anymore, such as polio. If, as vaccine espousers claim, we need these mass inoculations to protect our children from moribund illnesses because they may be brought into our country by foreigners, we would counter that it would be simpler and more cost effective to improve our monitoring of incomers, making sure they are vaccinated and unstricken by infection.

■ In order to really know which vaccines are safe and effective, we need to improve reporting of adverse vaccine-related episodes to VAERS.

This means efforts would have to be made to get physicians to pay careful attention to their patients' health post-inoculation. It would also be useful if the parents of children being given vaccines and others who were getting inoculated received forms on which they were mandated to mark the effects (if any) that appear after the shots. These would make a useful database which could be examined to study the typical side effects of different batches of vaccine.

Further, institutions that conduct mass vaccinations, such as the military and elementary schools, should encourage the reporting of side effects. Such organizations should look on themselves as partners in a scientific enterprise, trying to gather all relevant facts about the vaccine's character, rather than seeing themselves as transmission belts, who are carrying out orders from the medical establishment above.

■ Better testing procedures would help us weed out less promising vaccines before they went on the market.

We've seen repeated examples of vaccines that have been sped through the drug approval process because of putative threats of an epidemic. Even if such a fast-track procedure is occasionally justified, this doesn't mean a more careful screening couldn't be carried out even while the vaccine is being employed for emergency use.

Of utmost importance in testing is following the long-term effect of vaccines. We need to eschew current procedures, in which a one- or two-week period is considered sufficient time in which to note any unwarranted effects of the vaccination. Since we've seen that there are ill effects of vaccines that don't manifest until weeks or months after the dose was taken, drug trials must take more time and become observant of long-term as well as short-term problems. If the vaccine trials are done more scrupulously, we will have the assurance that vaccine injections that must be given are as safe as possible.

■ Another important step would be to raise the age of childhood inoculations.

"Vaccinations commences earlier in the United States than in any other country."[205] At the same time, our infant mortality rate, including deaths from such syndromes as SIDS for which there is no known cause, are the highest in the industrialized world. There may not be any connection, but we do know that tampering with a child's progressing physiology can wreak havoc.

In the words of the authors of *Vaccine Roulette*, "Babies and infants are physically too immature to be able to cope with the toxic load of the vaccines. Their bodies, and especially their brains, have not finished developing and maturing."[206] They comment further that a child has a more or less completely finished brain at age four or five. Before that time, it is under construction. "The cranial nerves are not fully insulated in early life, and it is this process of laying down the nerves' insulation which is very vulnerable to damage by vaccines."[207]

The injection of antigens into such a still-forming biological subject is chancy. It would seem wiser to wait and forestall the round of vaccines until the child is likely to meet many infectious agents as when he or she is about to enter primary school or has reached age three or four (at the earliest) and is going into daycare. Moreover, the immunizations should be staggered, with those least apt to produce ill effects given first. A careful monitoring of the side effects that appear in reaction to these more innocuous vaccines will alert the parents and physician to the child's level of tolerance. Of course, we are assuming that if any immunizations have to be given, they will only be those that are both necessary and relatively safe.

We have already suggested a division in how inoculations should be distributed, differentiating between those going to nursery school early and those staying at home till kindergarten. We argued separate immunization schedules should be set up for each group. Some will say it is not practical to fine-tune public health measures in this way. Nonetheless, such increased discrimination is the keystone of our understanding of how immunization should be re-focused.

■ We hold that mass inoculation programs should be dropped in favor of two discrete tacks. In normal times, there should be limited inoculation, targeted to those at high risk and given in a way that is responsive to the individual health of each recipient. During national emergencies when an engineered or natural epidemic appears, the vaccinated group should be amplified to include anyone who is related to a person coming down with the disease or who has been in a hazardous area.

Incao has encapsulated this strategy and its *raison d'être* in these terms:

> Use of vaccinations in medicine today is essentially a "shotgun" approach which ignores differences among individuals. In such an approach some individuals may be helped and some may be harmed.
>
> If medicine is to evolve in a healthy direction, we must learn to understand the particular characteristics of each individual, and we must learn how *to individualize* our treatments to be able to heal each unique human being.[208]

ARTIFICIALLY VERSUS NATURALLY BOOSTED IMMUNITY

The foregoing prescriptions are premised on the belief that *vaccines are not now and will never be our primary means of defense against infections.*

The reason vaccines cannot play the role of protector that many in public health expect them to play revolves around the nature of the new disease challenge we are facing.

We've seen that both pathogens created with terrorist action in mind and those that have naturally evolved into multi-drug resistant strains can maneuver their way around drugs that would destroy less developed versions of these germs. Since current vaccines (and other drugs) are largely aimed at destroying the more well-known, naturally occurring, unevolved disease types, they will have little impact on epidemics caused by more refined pathogens.

It's true that some work at Fort Detrick and other biological warfare facilities has created drugs to counteract what are projected as new disease agents. Cipro is a product of such research. However, the likelihood that what the laboratories guess is being made in terrorist strongholds (or, in other circumstances, what medical researchers think drug-resistant germs will be like) will coincide with what eventually will really appear is not very high.

But let's imagine that there is a snug fit and, for instance, our biodefense warriors correctly foresee the pathogens terrorist are concocting. Then they create suitable drugs to ward off these new germs. Think further. In order for drugs to have any effect on the illness-dispensing germs we sketched in Part 1 of our study, the drugs must be dispensed within a few days of infection. But these same germs generally cause symptoms that resemble those of flu or other mundane sicknesses and can easily be mistaken for these milder illnesses, thus delaying proper prophylaxis. This applies to antibiotics and other counteractive drugs.

As for vaccines, there is the time lag factor. These obviously, have to be given some time before a pathogen begins spreading. So if superb intelligence efforts and pharmaceutical finesse allowed us to learn of every bioweapon being spawned by terrorists and to match every germ with a vaccine, we would still have to develop a crash program, which would aim to inoculate our entire population every few months as new terrorist pathogens issued from their lab benches. But such a continuous dosing of the citizenry (or, at best, only those in big cities) with vaccines hardly seems feasible.

All in all, drugs are far from adequate instruments to circumvent outbreaks of new pathogens, although they will be able to reduce damage once an epidemic is identified. They cannot be counted on to guard us from these new threats.

Luckily, then, we have another and better line of defense, though it is one that is less discussed in traditional medical circles. *To shield ourselves from new pathogens we need to holistically and naturally ratchet up our immune systems.*

This recommendation can be easily misinterpreted. Under the old paradigm, boosting immunity simply consists of chocking the blood full of various antibodies. Usually this was done with pharmaceuticals. If the old instant cake mixes would tell the consumer, "Just add water"; the traditional medical practitioner's manner of building up a weakened immunity was to tell the patient, "Just add drugs." This is the rationale for vaccinations, after all.

The newer paradigm holds that disease is caused by a multitiered reaction between body, pathogen, and environment. If the body and its environment are not out of joint in the first place, a germ intruder will not cause much damage. In this view, healing does not simply mean killing off an intruder, but includes, beyond that, getting a person back up to peak immunity and seeing that the patient's environment is (if necessary) restructured so as to make it less stressful and unhealthy.

We will say more about this in our conclusion. What we want to discuss, in our second transition is the whole matter of paradigm shift, and in particular how people react under the stress it causes.

PASCAL AND THE BIRTH

OF A NEW PARADIGM

———

Near the beginning of this book we described a paradox in the life of Pascal. Here was a man who was in on the genesis of modern science, producing seminal works in both mathematics and physics. He suddenly changed course and began writing religious tracts. In both his chosen topic areas, he produced works of unquestionable genius.

The paradox here only appears if one remembers that in the West in the seventeenth century, math, physics and chemistry, while laying the foundation stones for the science we have now, were, at the same time, decisively undermining religion. Christianity would never be, as it had been in the Middle Ages, the sole ruler of the realm of thought. In the medieval period, religion had guided not only morality and worship, but hard science, from astronomy to physics to biology. Once the materialist viewpoint of Pascal, Descartes, Boyle, and other like-minded researchers had gained ground, though, forever after, science would sit on a second throne, co-equal monarch with religion of the intellectual world.

In starkest terms, the contradiction in Pascal's life is that in his first years (unconscious of the eventual effects of what he was doing) he was tearing the props out from under Catholicism, and in his last days, composing moving and novel defenses of the religion. How could one man over the course of a life stand at such opposite extremes?

A paradox can be used as a probing instrument since it concerns an event that shouldn't have happened, but did. If our predictions suggest the

———

opposite of what happened, then there must be something wrong with our suppositions. In this case, we have failed to see how what the French philosopher learned in the first half of his life by unfolding a new paradigm provided him with the ammunition he needed when he turned to his second major life activity, the revision of the Christian message so it was suitable for alignment with the century's new scientific outlook. This insight about the French thinker's life is laid out in an extraordinary book, *Discourse of the Fall: A Study of Pascal's* Pensées by Sara Melzer.

Now, you may have detected a logical difficulty with what I have already said. If Pascal was "unconscious of the eventual effects" of the rise of science on the church, then there would be no connection between his defense of religion and his previous actions, at least insofar as he personally didn't see any animus between science and the church. In fact, Pascal didn't seem to feel the new science was threatening to Catholicism. In writing about the church's clash with Galileo, he stated issues of fact—such as the Bible's view of astronomy versus that of the new physicists—would eventually be amicably settled without much harm to either side.

Yet, he did see a conflict in matters of overall world view. What he saw as a danger to the faith was this: The birth of science was demolishing the old paradigm in which God stood at the top of a great chain of being. If religion was to continue, it would need to reinsert itself into this new world view.

Pascal was the right man for the job of finding compatibilities between science and Christianity. The very penetration of his early work in math and physics helped him to see the full implications of the emergent scientific paradigm. This background allowed him to appreciate the extent of the re-creation that would be needed to redefine Christianity for the experimental age.

Let's look more specifically at how the old and new paradigms modeled reality.

> [The older] Renaissance paradigm [was] based on a finite, unified, hierarchically ordered world...all of whose parts have their place and meaning within the whole. The scientific revolution, however, revealed that the Renaissance paradigm was illusory by presenting a new one based on the infinite.[209]

The new way of looking at things saw nature as a system of mechanical devices. Everything from the solar system to animals, ran like a clock. The exception was humans who had souls, and thus belonged to a different order.

However, it was the boundlessness of the universe that science had revealed that was most disturbing to Pascal. He wrote, "*Le silence éternel de ces espaces infinis m'effraie.*" [The eternal silence of infinite space terrifies me.][210]

We can say briefly that Pascal in his work *Pensées* (notes for a treatise he never completed) was able to reconcile Catholicism with the emergent view by presenting a very different picture of God than the one that had him standing at the top of ladder of Renaissance cosmology.

For science, everything could be explained without God. Unchanging natural laws provided the program. Pascal agreed with this, but added, God wanted it this way. *The deity himself had created a Godless universe!* As Melzer puts it, "Pascal's God has withdrawn his presence from the scientific world as a punishment for the sins of humankind."[211]

In Pascal's own words: "Our religion…states that men lie in darkness, estranged from God, that He has hidden Himself from their knowledge, that such is the very name he takes in scripture, "the hidden God. [*Deus absconditus*]."[212]

The new paradigm did without a divinity, professly because God wanted it so. Science could teach humans their sinful nature. "By disclosing the distance between humans and the world, with its signs of God"—where the Renaissance had seen humans as very near to a world in which God was constantly meddling by performing miracles and doing other things for human advantage—"the modern world of the infinite can humble humans, thus reminding them of their fallen nature."[213] Thus, God's apparent absence did not mark his non-existence, but the fact that he was displeased with humankind. The Christian had to strive all the harder to find faith in such a seemingly deserted world.

We will come back to this in our conclusion, but let's move to a second point about Pascal and the new perspective. Not only did Pascal appreciate that the coming of a new paradigm would unsettle religion, but he saw that it would play havoc with morality.

On the most obvious level, it could be thought that if the material world didn't seem to have any need for God's intervention, then perhaps there really was no God. Without God, morality lost its linchpin. If God couldn't keep score on human behavior in order to mete out reward and punishment on Judgment Day, then, few would try to be good.

However, Pascal didn't think many people would go so far as turning atheists just because paradigms were in flux. What he did think was certain people would take advantage of the situation. These were the defenders of the status quo, who, in fighting a rearguard action to maintain the failing world view, provided rationalizations that would dangerously chip away at ethics. Before noting who this group was, we should state what bearing this has on our overall argument.

Many progressives have seen the new century as a time of deep malaise. Environmental destruction goes forward, sweatshops appear around the world, the Amazon rainforest is logged and burned, our food is tainted and tinkered with by biological engineers. All this is unsurprising to anyone conversant with the actions of governments and industry over the last few decades. What does seem new is the relative quiescence of citizens. Polls show, for example, that the vast majority of people in the United States want stronger environmental protection. Yet, as Bush weakens this protection to cater to big oil interests, little outrage is expressed in concrete action. Our contention is that part of the reason for this passivity is the confusion that flows through the populace at a time of paradigm shift.

(We might call this a "phase transition." In physics, this term refers to the unstable moment when matter is shifting from one mode of expression to another, as when H_2O is going from ice to liquid water.)

During a phase transition, reformers who want to preserve the old world view, know in their hearts that this view has formidable, perhaps disabling weaknesses. On the other hand, those who have cast in their lot with the new outlook still waver, hearing the constant belittling of this view by the establishment which controls the media, academia, and most other realms of information provision. They, too, often doubt themselves. In such a time, it is hard to act with unrestrained courage, because valor is based on calm assurance that what one is struggling for has unshakable validity. And in such times it is easy for equivocators to gain a hearing.

Pascal, also living in a period of intellectual upheaval, sought to describe the ploys of logic choppers to help his audience act more intelligently as it negotiated its way through trying circumstances. His analysis can be used to reflect on our own situation. Let's look at the background of his writings before seeing how it remains resonant today.

Within the Catholic church in France, Pascal was affiliated with a particular religious society called the Jansenists. In 1656, their spiritual leader, M. Arnauld, came under attack for heresy. The evidence against him was flimsy, and (in Pascal's eyes) had been trumped up by another Catholic society, the Jesuits, as a smear tactic. Arnauld had taken some swipes at the Jesuits in his books, and they wanted to get back at him.

In his *Provincial Letters*, Pascal set out to counter the charges of heresy, but as he fashioned his discussion, he began to look into the Jesuits' own practices, which seemed wanting. To him, the Jesuits, in their desire to be attractive to well-heeled, aristocratic parishioners, were willing to soften that creed. It was every church visitor's duty to make a confession of sins privately to a priest. The priest was then to give him a penance, prayers or other tasks that symbolized repentance. But, to Pascal, the Jesuits were relaxing the code of sins, excusing faults, such as dueling, which were much loved by the upper classes. They were even excusing the faults of the aristocrats' servants!

Most who read Pascal's witty and trenchant volume will be struck by some of the actions the Jesuits were allowing to pass muster. Pascal quotes, for instance, this passage where a Jesuit father is posed the following question about thievery, "If servants complain about their wages, can they increase them themselves by laying their hands on as much of their masters' property as they deem necessary to make the said wages equal their toil?" [214] The good father's answer, "They can do so in certain instances, as when…other servants of their kind earn more elsewhere."[215]

Shocking as such views may be, they are not of the essence. What is really intriguing (and resonant) in the *Provincial Letters* is when Pascal moves beyond individual examples to study the set of principles that stand behind them. One of these guiding assumptions is the principle of probable opinions. According to the imaginary Jesuit to whom Pascal talks, "An opinion [on such topics as whether so and so action is sinful or permissible] is called probable when it is founded on reasons of some importance."[216] Pascal comes back with the question of whether there could be only one probable opinion for each topic. But no.

> "You do not understand…. They [learned Jesuit doctors] very often do have different opinions; but that does not matter. Each one makes his own opinion probable and safe. Of course everyone knows that they do not all agree. And that is all to the good. On the contrary they almost never do agree…."
>
> "But, Father," I said, "one must be at a loss to choose then!"
>
> "Not at all," he said, "you have only to follow the more attractive opinion."[217]

Such a rule is tailor-made for a time of phase transition. It is a way to evade having to come down solidly for one perspective or another, as if all are equally valid.

Another innovative rationalization the Jesuits came up with was the idea of directing the intention, "which consists in setting up as the purpose of one's actions some lawful object."[218] Having an honest intention hardly seems blameworthy. But look at the way it is put to use. Again the reverend priest is talking:

> "That is how our Fathers have found a way to permit the acts of violence commonly practiced in the defense of honour [such as duels.] For it is only a question of deflecting one's intention from a desire for vengeance, which is criminal, and applying it to the desire to defend one's honour, which according to our Fathers is lawful. And so it is they fulfill all their duties to God and to men."
>
> [Pascal is then shocked by what lengths one is allowed to go by the church to defend honor. He ends, "So, you say,] one may have no qualms in killing…from behind or in ambush, some slanderer who is suing us."
>
> "Yes," said the Father, "but provided the intention is properly directed; you keep forgetting the main thing."[219]

This strategy would also provide a way to sidestep fully committing to one particular paradigm.

Perhaps, a anecdote will best show what I mean. Once I had been shopping in the Greenmarket at Union Square (in Manhattan). As I left, I ran smack dab into a man who had just completed my study group on vegetarianism. During the sessions he had presented himself as firmly committed to the vegan way. I guess that's why he turned beet red when he saw me. He had just emerged from McDonald's and held a juicy, half eaten Big Mac in one hand. The other held a sack full of its brothers. He said he thought one could eat meat occasionally as long as one was basically living a vegetarian lifestyle. I hope he doesn't have the same ideas about taking poison.

This man was straddling two lifestyles: carnivorous and herbivorous. And these time in with two paradigms, one believing poor health is due to invasive organisms, the other that it comes by way of collaboration between parasite and host, with the human host adopting an immune-weakening lifestyle.

Both these methods of finding excuses originated, we claim, as a way to let people hold on to the embattled paradigm. Rather than rethink Christian doctrine so as to make it compatible with the new world view, the Jesuits came up with ways that allowed one to vacillate between them (as well as to justify certain favored sins).

But let's move away from theology and see how the tense conditions during a phase transition occurred more directly in medicine.

PHILADELPHIA 1793

Abortive Phase Transition
in a Time of Cataclysm

———

1793 was also a year of paradigm clash. So, even as Philadelphia was sunken in a grim battle against the fever, its doctors were vociferously arguing over what was the best way to treat the sick, with the controversy seesawing between those who supported an older and newer world view.

The book that most clearly lays out the process of paradigm shift is Thomas Kuhn's *The Structure of Scientific Revolutions*.[220] However, profound as the book is, Kuhn presents a somewhat bloodless, schematic version of the orderly progress from one world view to another. As he explains, numerous anomalies accrue, which cannot be sorted out by the older problematic. Younger workers in the field are dissatisfied with this and cast about for a new way of looking at things; while their elders think of stopgap, ad hoc remedies to account for discrepancies. Then, a moment of revelation occurs. A group of scientists elaborate a new perspective, which gains the adherence of the younger set. Eventually, this new view wins the day.

If we look at what happened in Philadelphia, though, we see two major deviations from this outline.

To see what these are, we must begin by looking at Dr. Rush's methods. We've already mentioned Rush's progressive attempts to democratize medicine by calling for a simplification of the profession so anyone could be quickly made a physician. As of yet, though, we haven't looked at what Rush's treatments were.

———

In the eighteenth century, there was no set course of action for dealing with yellow fever, so as the epidemic worsened, "Rush tried all cures. He had begun in August with gentle purges and mild bleedings…and recommended cool air, cold drinks, low diet, and cold baths. This had resulted in nothing at all."[221] The doctor moved on through every suggested remedy, from doses of bark, wine, and aromatics, to the inducing of vomiting and wrapping the body in sheets dipped in vinegar. With the failure of each method, he spiraled deeper into feelings of defeatism. "Rush was frantic. 'Heaven alone bore witness to the anguish of my soul in this awful situation,' he wrote."[222]

Then one night, turning over an old MS on a yellow fever outbreak in Virginia in 1741 as described by Dr. John Mitchell, Rush underwent a powerful intellectual transformation. Mitchell's therapy for the stricken was violent purges of the bowels and a great use of bleeding. Rush thought:

> It was an extraordinary doctrine. Doctors had ever regarded their efforts as merely assistant to nature, yet Mitchell was blandly proclaiming the physician must domineer over nature, scorn her, command her.… Rush's imagination was immediately inflamed.[223]

Rush became a convert to and proselytizer for this method. The contentious doctor became scornful of other physicians who stayed with the tried-and-true milder treatments.

However, so far there may have been one misleading element in our account of Rush's breakthrough. It has not been made clear that Rush's revolutionary therapy was not a departure from the old paradigm. For all his intellectual excitement, he was simply making exaggerated use of conventional bloodletting and purging. A telltale clue to his traditionalism is that he arrived at his new idea, not according to observations made on the unwell but by reading.

Historian John Harvey Powell explains that eighteenth-century medicine took its cue from theory, not practice. "From the lecture hall at Edinburgh young graduates in medicine had gone out…taking with them the doctrines of Cullen and Monro.… They observed fevers through Cullen's eyes, wrote books about them in their teacher's words."[224]

If one wants to see the new paradigm struggling to be born, one would have to turn from the parlor of Dr. Rush to the charity hospital at Bush Hill. These facilities were under the direction of the French émigré, Dr. Jean Devèze. The two leading strings of Devèze's method were: (1) making treatment depend on observation of what works, and (2) varying the therapy in relation to each individual's constitution. He wrote:

> [1] Being in the habit of seeing the diseased, and to observe [I found] nature can alone guide the practitioner and render medicine a useful science.

> [2] Devèze thought it wrong to believe that] what succeeded well in one case, would have the same success in all others, though they appeared alike; because often an infinite number of hidden circumstances produced a change in the animal economy.[225]

This approach was unheralded. "Poor Devèze…has received little notice. He was an alien in an alien land. The fact that he saved lives where others failed could not overcome the suspicion in which he was held."[226] Nevertheless, this was the medicine of the future. Cures would be arrived at based on sound experiment where different methods were tried out, successes and failures tallied, and the best pursued. Moreover, in the best medicine, people would not be treated in the mass, but receive care personalized individual by individual.

Still, note how far the situation is from Kuhn's (admittedly) idealized case. While all the ink in Philadelphia's one remaining paper was spilled and all the medical quarreling centered on which of two versions of the dominant paradigm was the most viable, the new way of proceeding scientifically took place in an ignored backwater (the charity hospital), totally outside the whole public's and most of the medical profession's gaze.

And there is a second deviation from the ideal historical transformation. We've said that in Kuhnian thought the new world view grows in acceptance because it can explicate the reason behind anomalies that befuddle the elder theory. In medicine, then, we could say the new vision gained audience because it cured patients who were unaffected by traditional prophylactics.

So, let's ask: Was this the pattern in Philadelphia? Were the new methods outshining the old in gaining health and survival for the stricken?

Circumstances reversed what we would have expected.

Although it was recognized that Devèze had set the hospital to rights and was saving many patients, he still had a very high death rate because many patients put off coming to Bush Hill until they were beyond hope. Rush, on the other hand, constantly crowed over his success with the lancet (which was used in bleeding). He wrote, "The new medicine bears down all opposition," he wrote, and as Powell comments, "He formed the habit of saying, when called to a patient, 'You have nothing but yellow fever.'"[227]

Going forward, after the plague abated, Rush was celebrated as the savior of the city. He plumed himself, "To tell you of all the people who have been bled and purged out of the grave in our city, [by his treatment protocol] would require a book nearly as large as the Philadelphia directory."[228] This view was echoed in historical accounts, which uniformly credit Rush with medical miracles.

The problem is, we know now that his methods could not possibly have helped his patients. In truth, as Powell puts it,

> It is a still more difficult matter to explain how anyone he treated survived Rush's ministrations, particularly when we learn that he, like his contemporaries, thought there was about twice as much blood in the human body as there really was.[229]

Moreover, reading over the practices of Devèze, it can be seen that nothing he did was particularly valuable either. However, his open-minded dabbling with different therapies, and his attentive observation of these treatments' effects presaged the new medicine.

Thus we have the clash of two paradigms that were embodied in practices that were equally inept. Still, contrary to the ideal change during a phase transition, the older paradigm triumphed, even while it endangered the health of patients who only survived because of their own strong constitutions and immunity.

One last point. Previously, we brought up the concept of the default proto state. This arose in Philadelphia when the acting government decamped. A new one was recruited, literally, by taking out an ad in the newspaper, asking those who were interested in running the state to appear at City Hall the next day. We noted further that this proto government was futuristic, having a decentralized structure, a liberal power-sharing policy, and a reckless disregard for private property (seizing the Bush Hill property, for example, without anyone's permission). Some of the newly instituted methods, such as the employment of African-Americans in leadership positions, would not become common practice in the United States until 175 years later; others, such as the widespread distribution of power to anyone who wanted to participate, never.

We emphasized, also, this proto state was an emergency formation, meant and understood to be a way to maintain minimal but essential activities (burials, hospitals, care of orphans, and so on) during an interregnum.

(By the way, this interregnum created problems for the federal government as well. When Washington wanted to move the federal government to Germantown, his vice president, Adams, objected that this would be breaking the Constitution and would represent a usurpation of power.)

When the plague died down, the old guard with its bureaucratic procedures was welcomed back.

We've said all that. But, can we imagine for a moment a counterfactual situation. We want to wonder why the temporary holders of office did not try to prolong their control. Such things have happened before.

A glance at history will show that Philadelphia's interim government had no interest in staying longer than necessary. Why is that? We think it is because *what one can imagine determines how one acts.* To envision the type of government they improvised as of lasting value would demand their orient their thought within a new world view that was more widely democratic and experimentally based than the one obtaining at the time. The barest tracings of this new perspective are visible in Devèze's tentative probings.

We hold that the quick reversion to a less wieldy, less representative state form was no tragedy; because without a relatively explicit new paradigm standing under the radical changes they were making, they would find little support for the new dispensation in the society or in their own hearts.

Yet, there is a rich paradox in this. What Devèze was doing and what the interim city governors were doing could not be sustained outside of a crisis because a new perspective had not been created to give their efforts credibility. Yet, how is it that they acted as they did? How could they have created this unprecedented structure unless they had some vague premonition of a new way of life?

NATURE OF THE EMERGENT
MEDICAL PARADIGM

———

We have harped on the fact that earlier periods of phase transition can give some guidance to our historical situation. We have presented the experience of Pascal with those who tried to hold back the irresistible move to a scientific world outlook by temporizing and the experience of the Philadelphia doctors as they struggled with yellow fever as so many mirrors of our own unstable time.

One thing lacking in all this has been a very precise discussion of new health paradigm. Let's spend a few minutes on this topic. We simply want to say that the new viewpoint on health emphasizes all-inclusiveness. As opposed to traditional medicine, which, when confronted with an infectious disease, goes all out to kill the pathogen, but pays desultory attention to conditions that made the patient susceptible in the first place; alternative care would not only act to cure the infection, but try to place the incursion of illness into a wider perspective. The alternative practitioner would survey the patient's physical, mental, and *social* climate in order to discover if any factors had contributed to susceptibility.

By way of illustration, let's imagine, God forbid, a woman was infected with anthrax after a terrorist attack. In this case, while others showed no signs of illness, she was made gravely ill, though, fortunately, with alternative treatment, she pulled through. After recovery, on consulting her practitioner, the patient would be asked to engage in preventive measures to ensure that if in the unlikely possibility she was caught in a second bioter-rorism incident, she would not succumb to the infection so easily. These measures would be multi-directional.

Physically, she would boost her immune system, using some of the recommendations found in this book or elsewhere. She would also modify her life, if necessary, in order to fill it with health-enhancing practices, in-cluding eating a vegetarian diet and exercising.

Mentally, she would ready herself for the possibility of another high-stress event, such as being infected with a dangerous germ, by learning relaxation techniques, which help one to center during trying periods. Moreover, she would fortify her intellect by keeping informed on medical trends as well as about the appearance of new pathogens.

Socially, she would continue her perusal of contemporary reports, looking beyond the immediate dangers posed by new pathogens into the reasons, fixed in the structure of global society, they are constantly being re-leased. She would note in the United States the undersupport of public health, and in the world, the inequality, injustice, and poverty that nurture the growth of terrorism. Selecting the area of controversy that she felt most passionate about, she would join an organization acting to improve society. Her participation would not only help her individually, for it is health en-hancing to work with others for positive goals, but make the world a place less liable to harbor new infections.

Integrating these elements, our imagined character would have changed from what she was at first, a hapless sufferer from the buffetings of the world, to what she was after improving her immunity, attitude, and activism: some-one who decides to redefine herself and her surroundings. Obviously, any reader can also take this route. Let's look at this tripartite quest in all detail.

PART III

NATURAL WAYS TO WARD OFF

THE INCURSION OF NEW GERMS

W e won't hide the fact that in its advisory on bioterrorism, the director of the National Center for Complementary and Alternative Medicine (NCCAM), Stephen Strauss, MD, came down firmly against any reliance on alternative treatments for protection. Before glancing at what he had to say, though, remember the NCCAM is a government agency under the direction of the National Institutes of Health. Its job is not to espouse alternative healing but to check the claims of untraditional practices.

Before a House subcommittee, Strauss stated,

> While augmenting one's natural healing powers [through alternative therapies] may prove beneficial for some illnesses...there is no scientific basis to believe that this approach would be of much value in the context of virulent diseases incited by biological weapons.... Diseases like anthrax, smallpox, and tularemia exceed one's innate immunity to control them, and progress too rapidly for specific and protective antibody and lymphocyte responses to evolve. Simply stated, they can kill us before we can arm ourselves fully to defend against them.[1]

One thing you can say for Strauss, he goes right to the nub of the disagreement between traditional and alternative treatment. From the non-traditional perspective we adopt, the central component of an intelligent response to the danger of new disease incursion is using natural means to make individuals' immunity more flexible and vigorous. Better immunity primes the body in advance to counter unexpected pathogen intrusion. We can allow Strauss some basis for his opinion, in that these new germs are of unprecedented virulence. We should recognize further that when one is actually made ill by a new germ, traditional techniques generally work best, particularly in that such methods have been developed to be particularly attuned to crises. This last point should clue us in to the real thrust of Strauss's argument. No one is saying, for instance, to begin boosting one's immunity *after one has contracted smallpox.* So any disputes that may arise between alternative and conventional treatment will only be about prevention, and it is alternative preventives that Strauss disparages.

The alternative healer says immune boosting is the way to go to face these new biological dangers. The traditional practitioner looks to vaccines and other drugs as the answer. Before proceeding to our recommendations for immune system enhancement, let us reiterate a few facts that have been established thus far.

FACT: Aside from anthrax, smallpox, and a few other illnesses, which have at least some viable prophylactics, **there are no vaccines, antibiotics, antivirals or other treatments against most the diseases on the CDC's list of probable terrorist bio-agents. Multi-drug-resistant germs are by definition ones that don't respond to known cures.**

Thus, in relation to most of the diseases, one either crosses one's fingers and does nothing while waiting for pharmaceutical companies to come up with preventives or treatments or one follows the alternative way to bolster immunity.

FACT: If the World Trade Center attack taught us anything, **it is that effective terrorists do the unexpected. Surprise is key to their strategy. In consequence, we can never be sure we are vaccinating or creating stores of antibiotics and anti-pathogens for the right germs.**

Just as the French military, in a famous phrase, was characterized as being experts in "fighting the last war," so our biological defense are probably great at "preparing for the last terrorist outrage." Let's put it this way. Given that tremendous publicity and laudable research are now going into guarding our country against terrorists armed with anthrax and (to a less extent) smallpox, is it probable that the next round of incidents will involve either of these pathogens?

Remember further that even when drugs are created that anticipate new pathogens, such as Cipro, which was developed as a countermeasure against a souped-up anthrax, they can easily be outfoxed. Terrorists might, for example, combine anthrax with another germ or toxin, creating a Russian doll cocktail. Such concoctions, as we've mentioned, are state of the art for bioterrorists. In the case of such surprises, the traditional medical arsenal would be useless. Building an individual's immunity at least offers some hope of disease prevention.

FACT: **No disease spreads to everyone exposed or proves fatal to everyone who catches it.** You'll remember that an outbreak is considered major when, as in the 1793 Philadelphia yellow fever epidemic, 20 percent of the population die. In all cases, even with Ebola and the other most powerful germs, a goodly percentage of the affected are sickened, then recover. Further, without doubt, those who die or recover are not the total number who were infected. Some, in the case of cholera, for example, imbibe the germ through water, or, for yellow fever, are bitten by carrier mosquitoes, but manage to kill the pathogen before it causes any ill effects. Putting together those who recover and those who eliminate the germ before it can spread, we can say that one reason behind people pulling through is that they have strong immune systems. Other reasons would be they received a smaller dose of the germ or a less virulent form; but there are certainly cases where a healthy immunity helped protect the infected. For this percentage, immune enhancement paid off.

FACT: **In most cases, as we will elaborate, even if alternative treatments may not be as surefire as vaccines and other traditional medical procedures (as far as conventional means work), they are also beset with few or none of the devastating side effects that accompany mainstream drugs and therapies.**
As we've seen, antibiotics, while life-saving when correctly taken, can do more harm than good when used indiscriminately by spurring the growth of resistant bacteria and weakening the immune system thus rendering it more prone to secondary and recurrent infections. For people in whom exposure is likely but not proven or certain high-risk categories, such as pregnant women, young children, the elderly, or people with known allergies, the dangers of a high-dose, long-course antibiotic therapy may offset its potential benefits.

If one is contemplating preventive measures in the face of newly emergent pathogens, concerns for side effects may make one put immune system improvement at the top of one's list. Vaccinations may go at the bottom.

Let's see how you would go about bolstering your immunity as well as taking other steps to round out a healthy, germ-resistant life.

Of course, the first thing to do to escape infections is to stay away from contaminated areas or, if one is in such an area, to reduce exposure. The two main things determining the impact of a chemical or biological weapon are level of exposure and host immunity. Preventive measures to reduce level of exposure would be the use of air purifiers with high HEPA ratings; wearing of protective garments, such as gloves; cleanliness and antisepsis, and departure from areas of suspected contamination

As for the second determinant, we have to empower our immune system by detoxification, deacidification, de-stressing, and using herbs and nutrients with immune-boosting properties. We will go through each of these in turn. Before this, it will be worth our time to say a few general things about nutrition in general. (We saw that according to McKeown, it was better nutrition, not public health or any other measure, that was responsible for near elimination of most of the epidemic diseases of the nineteenth century.) After our study of immune enhancement, we will say a few words about alternative practices, such as homeopathy, which have something to contribute to improving our existence. In our conclusion, we will talk about social factors of health.

Diet

E ating right is the pivot around which a wholesome life revolves. It wouldn't do much good to swallow all kinds of herbs and vitamins if, at the same time, one chowed down every night at Winky Burgers. A good diet lays the foundation for immune health, which supplements then build on.

From my own point of view as a vegetarian, the first move to proper nutrition is to stop eating meat. However, rather than discuss the reasons and benefits of such a course, which I have explained at length in other works, let's look at what many would consider the more temperate advice of Dr. Garth Nicolson. He does not totally disavow meat eating, but does see eye to eye with me on both what foods are to be utterly avoided and which foods should serve as centerpieces to a reasonable eating plan.

Dr. Nicolson and his medical group have worked consistently with patients who suffer from Gulf War Syndrome and other chronic immune-weakened conditions. He has seen patients make turnarounds in fighting these ailments once they begin healthy eating. On the down side, he says, "We have found that patients who refuse to change their dietary habits usually do not recover."[2]

Nicolson's recommendations are not only applicable to those suffering from debilitating diseases, but were devised to be generally useful to those who want to firm up their overall immunity. Many of his suggestions derive from his knowledge of how specific foods either suppress or give ammunition to the growth of infectious agents.

For instance, the food and beverages that he feels are no-no's are ones that are promoters of pathogen activity, while many foods he thinks should be consumed help us wage war on germs. Briefly stated, here are his do's and don't's.

AVOID

SUGAR

The bulk of invasive germs dote on sugar. "Most pathogenic or disease-causing microorganisms require simple sugars, so high-sugar diets actually stimulate their proliferation."[3]

CAFFEINE

Colas, coffee, tea, chocolate, and other caffeine-bearing drinks and foods also further the advance of unwanted microorganisms. A steady intake of coffee or other caffeine-heavy items will alter blood properties and weaken immune trajectories.

MILK PRODUCTS

Besides being strong allergens, which trigger allergic reactions in many people, these products, from cheese to cow milk, encourage the growth of fungi and yeast. Milk contains high amounts of fat and sugar, neither of which is helpful in a diet.

CANNED FOODS

To prepare such foods for a long shelf life in the supermarket, these substances must be riddled with salts, nitrates, and preservatives. These additives irritate the bowel lining, can lead to high blood pressure, and, in some cases, have been identified as carcinogens.

STARCHY FOODS

These do not have to be totally shunned, but large amounts in the diet are counterproductive. Starch is gradually broken down in the body into the simple sugars, which give a leg up to invading germs. Too much pasta and bread in one's food plan is, thus, something to be steered away from.

ALCOHOL

Beer, wine, and many alcoholic drinks contain large doses of sugar. Moreover, alcohol, like starch but at a faster rate, converts to sugar once it has been consumed. This substance hurts both the gastrointestinal lining and the threads of the nervous system.

YEAST

Too much yeast in the diet "add[s] to the overall burden of yeast and fungi in your gut."[4] Some of the yeast and fungi found in the gastrointestinal system are beneficial, but other forms are disease-causing. Yeast will indiscriminatingly contribute to the growth of both.

EMBRACE

VEGETABLES AND FRUIT

These should be the your main course. Vegetables contain vitamins, minerals, phytochemicals, and fiber. The first three promote immune strength and the last (as will be noted in our next point) helps remove harmful bacteria from the gut. Pathogenic bacteria and fungi need sugars and lipids to proliferate, and since vegetables provide none, a diet high in vegetables starves these intruders. Along with fiber, vegetables help push food through the intestines, "moving pathogenic bacteria and fungi through your gut" for quick elimination.[5] To repeat, vegetables are filled with natural medicines and tonics of high quality; so, while providing nutrition, they also contribute to overall physical well being.

DIETARY FIBER

Bacteria love to sit and ferment in the gut. So frequent bowel movements are needed to keep them in check by pushing undigested food and the bacteria themselves out of the intestines. Fiber is found not only in fruit and vegetables but in grains, cereals, nuts, and seeds. As Leo Galland, MD, comments, "High fiber diets support the growth of Lactobacilli and other friendly flora in the large intestine and inhibit the ability of disease causing bacteria and parasites to attach themselves to the intestinal wall."[6]

WATER AND JUICE

Ironically enough, for all Americans' vaunted overconsumption, they don't drink enough water. As we've seen, food and drink do not only provide nutrients and immune enhancer, but they are involved in flow-through, the continual flushing of the system that keeps it healthy. Majid Ali, MD, speaking more technically, notes that excessive acidity and oxidativeness, both conditions being manifestation of stress and the impact of environmental pollutants, fill the body with toxins. "The simplest and most effective measure for reducing...this stress is to dilute and eliminate the acidotic—and oxidative—molecules with increased fluid intake."[7]

Dr. Majid Ali recommends drinking eight glasses of water or juice a day. Natural fruit and vegetable juices combine the flushing qualities of water with the nutritiousness of the plant foods.

THE RIGHT OILS

Ali also notes that using cold-pressed oils (a.k.a., unrefined oils) is essential to a good diet. Refined, commercially processed oils use chemicals or solvents to remove the oil from the bean, seed or other source. This method strips the oil of vitamin E and other nourishing elements. Cold pressed oils are made, as the name implies, by pressing down on the source to squeeze out the oil. No chemicals or solvents are involved.

Ali recommends rotating the following oils: extra virgin olive oil, flaxseed oil, sesame oil, grapeseed oil, avocado oil, pumpkin oil, safflower oil, canola oil, garlic oil, and cod liver oil.

Oils are needed by the body to construct cell membranes, and are useful in metabolism whereby fats are broken down for use in the body's energy exchange patterns.

HERBS AND SPICES

Most of the herbs and spices we now use for seasoning were originally valued as preservatives, which means they kept food from deteriorating by stopping the proliferation of germs. Some of the herbs and spices most recognized for their healing capacities are: garlic, which in many studies has demonstrated it can provide protection against assorted bacteria, fungi, parasites, and viruses; turmeric, which eliminates bacteria that cause intestinal gas as well as countering inflammation; and ginger, which protects the stomach lining and kills intestinal parasites.[8]

Thus a good diet feeds, flushes, and medicates the body. Nicolson feels one should divide one's food intake in this way. Two-thirds should be vegetables and fruits, with the emphasis on the former, since "most fruits contain sugars and acids, so they must be used in moderation."[9] This would include not only green, orange, and yellow vegetables but juices made from them. The remaining third of the diet should be divided between starches, such as grains, rice, and bread; and protein. Although Nicolson would allow non-red meat in this final category, I would emphasize that one can get fully adequate protein simply by consuming a proper mix of beans, nuts, seeds, tofu, and grains.

However, establishing a good eating plan may not be enough to get your body in tiptop shape in the dietary area. Many people, because of overindulgence in the don'ts or due to unusual stress and other immune-weakening events, need something of a physical and mental overhaul. When they are in this condition, the body needs to be rid of toxins and acidity, and the mind of stress before a renovated diet plan will lead to optimum health and a super immune system. Let's see what steps can be taken to get the body in its best working order.

Detoxification

Toxins accumulated in the body impair the function of living cells, impose excessive workload to the detoxification systems, and reduce the efficiency of the immune system. To rev up energy levels and potentiate immunity, it is crucial to begin eliminating stored toxins from the body. To do so, the sensible method is to work with the body's active detoxification and elimination systems, which are, basically, the gastrointestinal tract, the liver, the lymphatic system, the skin, the lungs, and the kidneys.

THE GASTROINTESTINAL TRACT

The gastrointestinal tract processes and eliminates toxins ingested through food and water. Its inner cavity is inhabited by trillions of beneficial microorganisms, which support its proper functioning. The most important of the bacteria in the intestine are *Lactobacillus acidophilus* and *Bifidobacterium bifidum*. Intestinal bacteria produce vitamins and nutrients that are absorbed through the bloodstream, metabolize toxins, help maintain the integrity of the intestinal lining so that it is less permeable to toxins, and inhibit the growth of disease-producing organisms. To keep this part of the detoxifying system in good working order, you need to eat foods that will keep digestion moving at a good clip and that bolsters beneficial bacteria. Some food that can be eaten contains beneficial gut bacteria, which, once consumed, are transferred to one's own system.

FIBER

A moment ago we talked about the significance of fiber in the diet, showing then its protective and nurturing qualities. We need to be even more specific about the part it plays in aiding toxic elimination in the gastrointestinal region.

Fiber can be soluble or insoluble in water.

Soluble fiber forms a thick gel. Fruit pectins, mucillages, and hemicelluloses, such as oat bran, are types of soluble fiber. This fiber is fermented in the gut, forming short-chain fatty acids. These acids provide multiple benefits. They feed the intestinal cells, inhibit the growth of harmful bacteria and yeasts, and decrease cholesterol formation in the liver, thus lowering cholesterol blood levels.

Insoluble fiber does not dissolve in water, but rather binds to it, thickening its mass in a way that promotes bowel movements. Thus, while soluble fiber works to rid us of intrusive germs and and beef up the action of positive microorganism, insoluble fiber, such as wheat bran, aids in the quicker transit of materials through the gut, thus speeding the elimination of toxins in waste.

A diet rich in fiber is extremely important to optimal health. If you only have a bowel movement a day and eat three times a day, you have build-ups of toxins in your intestine, and need to start detoxifying. Constipation is associated with low fiber intake. When we increase the amount of fiber we eat, we increase our bowel movements.

For detoxification of the gastrointestinal tract, the following regimen is recommended. Start by taking a fiber product, such as psyllium husks and flax seeds, morning and night. Take one to two teaspoons of powdered psyllium husks or one to two tablespoons of soaked or ground flax seeds daily. Mix the product with good water or juice and have it on an empty stomach. Drink plenty of water with it, as water is needed to swell the fiber, creating bulk in the intestinal tract. The fiber will work through your intestine like a broom, cleaning out old debris and will help reestablish a healthy intestinal flora. It's important to have at least two bowel movements a day.

ENEMAS AND COLONICS

To help the elimination of old junk that has remained stuck in the intestinal lining, you may add enemas and colonics. Enemas can be included as part of a detoxification program, but should not be used on a regular basis as they could alter intestinal flora and create addiction. Colonic irrigations use warm filtered water to remove buildups of waste and toxins accumulated in the intestinal wall. The procedure lasts forty-five minutes to an hour, and can lead to impressive cleansing results.

PROBIOTICS

Aside from cleaning the gut and giving support to vital, symbiotic bacteria that reside there, for a thoroughgoing detoxification, it is also necessary to eat foods that contain the probiotic (health-nurturing), friendly bacteria.

Consuming live yogurt or sauerkraut is one way of supplementing the diet with lactobacilli. Many commercially available yogurts do not contain live cultures; so before purchasing them make sure they have not been heat-treated after the bacterial cultures are added. Also make sure your yogurt comes from organic milk, as the antibiotics, vaccines, hormones, and pesticides given to cows all get concentrated in milk.

Unpasteurized sauerkraut is another excellent source of friendly bacteria. It contains *L. plantarum*, a normal inhabitant of the human intestine.

Probiotics can also be obtained in nutritional supplements. The best brands incorporate FOS (fructooligosaccharides), short-chain sugars that feed friendly bacteria and discourage the growth of undesirable species. A high quality commercial preparation provides for an infusion of friendly bacteria that will be longer lasting than the colonization of bacteria that comes from simply eating yogurt. This is because yogurt is generally prepared with *L. bulgaricus* and *Streptococcus thermophilus*, bacteria that disappear from the gastrointestinal tract rather quickly.

Take your bacterial supplement on an empty stomach, at least one hour before a meal or two hours after. It is especially important to take probiotics during and after antibiotic therapy, at a dosage of at least 15–20 billion organisms.

THE LIVER

The gastrointestinal tract specializes in two things, breaking down food so that its useful nutrients can be parceled out among the body's cells and eliminating toxins and unfriendly germs that have come in with that food. The liver, by contrast, has only one major role in relation to utilizing incoming matter: detoxification of the blood. The liver is the body's master cleanser, designed to filter and eliminate impurities from the blood that are absorbed from the gastrointestinal tract, the lungs, and the skin, or produced by the body's metabolism. The liver effectively removes bacteria, antigen-antibody complexes, endotoxins, and cell debris from circulation. It detoxifies and excretes through the bile such toxins as drugs, hormones and pesticides. Aside from doing this, like many other internal organs, such as the thymus, the liver is a factory, mass-producing, storing, synthesizing, and distributing vitamins, nutrients, and hormone precursors throughout the body. It also is involved in the manufacture of lymph, a fluid which transports fat-soluble nutrients around the body and drains cellular waste and harmful microorganisms that have escaped the bloodstream.

In its significant role as detoxifier, the liver is often called upon to take up the slack when the gastrointestinal system is not pulling its weight. An increase in the amount of toxins that enter into the gut, coupled with a decrease in the bowel's ability to eliminate such toxins, will force the liver to take on an extra work load. When too much work is placed upon the liver, its ability to detoxify will be progressively compromised, and symptoms such as fatigue, difficulty in concentration, headaches, skin problems, gastrointestinal disturbances, menstrual disorders, and allergies, to name a few, will develop. Luckily, the liver has incredible regenerating abilities, and simple lifestyle changes and beneficial practices can restore liver function to its optimal ability.

To put an over-stressed liver back on track, the first thing to do is to reduce the intake of toxins in the body. Eating organic food, drinking pure water, reducing the intake of processed foods, caffeine, sugar, and saturated, polyunsaturated, and hydrogenated fats will take a big burden off your liver. In other words, the first move in liver enhancement is to follow the eating prescriptions we laid out at the head of this section.

Consuming good quality fats such as monounsaturated oils and omega-3 essential fatty acids will improve the functioning of the liver. These fats can be obtained via flax oil, olive oil, and natural oils present in raw nuts and seeds as well as in cold-water fatty fish, such as tuna and salmon.

A good diet can be supplemented with milk thistle (*Sylibum marianum*), an herb with a long history of use as liver remedy. Research has shown that its active ingredient, silymarin, protects liver cells from damage induced by different types of toxins, including alcohol, industrial poisons, and even from poisoning with *Amanita phalloides*, a mushroom that contains one of the most potent liver toxins known. Milk thistle is also capable of stimulating regeneration of already damaged liver cells. Supplements with standardized silymarin content offer the greatest protection.

While consumption of these foods and herbs support normal liver function, to cleanse the liver one can rely on an old-time recipe prescribed by naturopathic physicians. The liver and gall bladder flush is a beverage made with citrus fruits, oil and pungent herbs that stimulates the production and secretion of bile from the liver and the gallbladder, facilitating the dumping of stored toxins into the gastrointestinal tract, from which they will be summarily eliminated.

LIVER AND GALL BLADDER FLUSH

In a blender mix together:

> Juice of 1 sweet grapefruit
> Juice of 1 or 2 lemons or limes
> 2 tablespoons of extra virgin olive oil
> 1 inch of ginger root or 1 clove of raw garlic
> Pinch of cayenne pepper

Drink the flush on an empty stomach first thing in the morning. Do not eat any solid food for the next two to three hours.

In addition to the flush, you can increase intake of foods that stimulate liver function. Fresh, bitter, dark green vegetables stimulate the flow of bile, and therefore help cleanse the liver and improve digestion. They can be eaten raw in salads, or slightly steamed or sautéed.

LIVER CLEANSING FOODS

> Arugula
> Carrots
> Collard greens
> Dandelion
> Endive
> Kale
> Mustard greens
> Parsley
> Watercress

THE LYMPHATIC SYSTEM

Above, we briefly characterized the lymph fluid. It is less known to the public than blood, but like the blood is the core of its own circulatory system. Where blood in its transport role takes oxygen and nutrients to the cells, lymph, made up of plasma and lymphocytes, takes cellular waste and microorganisms through the filtering system of the lymph nodes and eventually to the heart. The nodes are part of the lymphatic system, which is an extensive network of lymph vessels that run parallel to the blood vessels and reach almost every cell in the body. Scattered throughout the lymphatic system are groups of small, bean-shaped organs, called lymph nodes, inhabited by lymphocytes, which are cells of the immune system that trap and kill microorganisms. The lymph nodes process the wastes and then these are emptied into the blood, where they are eliminated by the liver, the kidneys, and the large intestine. When the lymph system is sluggish, stagnation occurs, cellular waste backs up, so microorganisms will have more chances of escaping immune surveillance, and infections are more likely to occur. This part of the body's detoxification also has to be kept in fighting trim.

Exercise, massage and dry skin brushing are three ways to assure tiptop lymphatic function.

EXERCISE

Unlike the blood, which is automatically pumped by the heart, lymph is set going by the movements of all muscles. When we exercise, the lymph gets moved throughout the body so it can get on with its work of removing toxins. When we take deep breaths, we further stimulate the flow of lymph by moving the diaphragm up and down, which creates a pumping action that pushes the lymph from the main lymphatic duct, located right behind the chest bone, into the bloodstream.

Research has shown that moderate exercise increases the function of the immune system. Any activity that gets you moving is beneficial. Ideally, you should do forty minutes of aerobic exercise three to five times a week. These workouts can be supplemented by the simpler expedient of taking three consecutive deep inhalations and holding your breath for a few seconds before exhaling. This will open the lymphatic duct, allowing the dumping of lymph into the blood.

MASSAGE

While exercise is a necessary but vigorous way to get the lymph flowing, a more restful method to accomplish this needed task is whole body massage. Ideally, during detoxification, you should treat yourself to a massage at least twice a week.

If this is unfeasible, you can massage yourself using a simple scrubbing technique.

HOT TOWEL SCRUB

Fill a basin with very hot water. Dig a small cotton towel in it and wring it to remove excess water. Rub the cloth vigorously on one foot until it turns rosy. Dig the cloth into the water again and start working on your calf, proceed with the thigh and other leg working your way up toward the heart. Continue rubbing down the rest of your body, and lastly rest it on your face, so the heat opens the pores. This simple technique takes five to ten minutes to do and will boost the lymphatic system, situated just beneath the skin surface.

DRY SKIN BRUSHING

Another type of rubbing that is useful in stimulating the lymphatic system involves the use of a brush.

Use a natural bristle brush. The body should be dry and naked, and the brush should be swept with long, smooth strokes in the direction of the heart along the entire body, except the face. Do not apply too much pressure on the brush nor make rotary movements. Just sweep it from feet to waist, from hands to shoulders, down the neck, across the shoulders, down the back and torso, and up the belly and buttocks.

This massage stimulates both the lymph system and the superficial blood circulation and enhances drainage of waste material from tissues. Daily skin brushing also exfoliates dead skin cells, leaving the skin smooth and hydrated while making you feel invigorated.

We might add that exercise, massage, and brushing not only give impetus to the lymphatic system but invigorate another major site of detoxification, the skin.

THE SKIN

Approximately 25 percent of the body's waste products are eliminated through the skin, and many environmental pollutants find their way out through this organ. This is why sweating plays such an important role in detoxification. If the ability of other elimination organs to remove waste is impaired, the skin will try to compensate by expelling toxins from the body. Acne or abscesses may result.

The skin also directly absorbs nutrients and toxins, so beware of what you put on it. Buy only personal care products made with natural ingredients that you can find at your local health food store.

Since exercise makes us sweat, while it is firming muscles, increasing metabolism, and stimulating lymph flow, it is a fine assister of the skin in its eliminative processes. Other, less vigorous ways to draw toxins through the skin are saunas and hot bathes.

SAUNAS

Skin cleanses have been performed throughout the centuries by many cultures in saunas, steambaths, and sweat lodges. The heat generated in saunas opens the skin pores and induces perspiration, promoting elimination of the backlog of waste and poisons accumulated in the fatty tissue below the skin surface.

If you are pregnant or suffer from cardiovascular disease, do not use saunas or steam baths without consulting your health practitioner. Otherwise, when intent on detoxification, use saunas or steambaths twice a week. The temperature should allow you to work up a moderate sweat in ten to fifteen minutes, and should allow you to stay in for forty-five to sixty minutes altogether, allowing for brief intermissions. Three fifteen- to twenty-minute sessions, interrupted by cold showers, provide excellent detoxification benefits. Drink plenty of water during and after your sauna. You can spike the water with chlorophyll to further stimulate toxin elimination. When engaged in a heavy sauna regimen, take mineral supplements, seeing as heavy sweating promotes mineral loss as well as the flushing out of toxins.

BATHS

Another simple way to increase waste elimination through the skin is to take hot water baths. Hot water opens up the skin pores and draws toxins to the skin surface, and, as the water cools, it pulls them out of the skin into the water. However, do not remain in the tub for more than twenty minutes.

Adding alkaline salts into the water further increases cleansing. Epsom salts (magnesium sulfate), baking soda (sodium bicarbonate), and Dead Sea salts can be added to the water bath, and will leave your skin smooth and soft. Below are two mixtures that help with the skin cleansing offered by a hot bath.

MIXED SALT BATH FORMULA

1/2 cup sea salts (purchased at the health food store)
1 cup baking soda
1/2 cup Epsom salts
1 to 2 tablespoons of olive or sesame oil per bath

Combine the salts in a container and pour into the bath while the tub is filling. Add one to two tablespoons of olive or sesame oil to keep your skin from drying out. You can add your essential oils of choice.

SALT AND SODA BATH FORMULA

1 cup baking soda
1 cup Epsom salts (or coarse salt or sea salt)

Add to the bath and soak for 15 minutes, sponging your face with a cloth while soaking.

THE LUNGS

We've all heard that the average human only uses a small portion of available brain cells in the course of his or her life. Whether that idea is true or not, what is true, but not as well known, is that the average person only uses a limited portion of his or her lung capacity in breathing. If the lung is not fully expanded, this, too, weakens the body's detoxification capacity. Remember that the lungs not only draw in oxygen, but expel waste carbon dioxide produced by cell metabolism.

All of us are familiar with the feeling we get when we are in the woods, mountains, or other natural setting and spontaneously start expanding our chest to get more fresh air. We usually feel an energy surge, not only due to the increase in oxygen, but because of the breathing out of toxins. Stress evaporates, the mind relaxes, and our mood improves.

Full breathing helps the lung cleanse from mucus build-up and supports the activity of immune cells against bacteria, viruses, allergens, and pollutants that enter through the respiratory system. In addition, proper breathing helps the body cleanse by increasing blood oxygen and decreasing blood carbon dioxide.

To get the lungs to do their utmost in detoxifying, it is important to combine a good diet with deep breathing exercises.

DIET

We've already outlined the optimal diet, but here we need to stress the elimination of foods that spur mucus production. Mucus is a slimy substance secreted in the respiratory system to coat and protect the throat, lungs, mouth, and other linings. However, too much of a good thing, too much mucus, that is, can clog and interfere with normal breathing processes; so, it is important to avoid mucus-forming foods, such as dairy and flour products, processed foods, and sugar. To cut down on already-existent mucus congestion, sip hot water with lemon and drink plenty of water.

Beyond that, lung cleansing can be aided by eating foods that are especially rich in chlorophyll, such as chlorella, spirulina, and barley grass.

DEEP BREATHING

If you watch how a baby breathes, you'll learn how to breathe properly. When we are born, we know instinctively how to deep breathe, but with time we have replaced this knowledge with shallow breathing. To maximize the elimination of toxic gases as well as to increase the inflow of vitalizing oxygen, we need to re-learn how to breathe.

DEEP BREATHING EXERCISE

Put both hands on your belly and take a deep breath. Expand the diaphragm down into your abdomen, letting your chest expand along with it. If you see your belly pushing your hands out, it means you are using your diaphragm to breathe. Hold the breath for a comfortable amount of time, before starting slowly exhaling. Continue breathing this way for a few minutes.

At the beginning of this exercise you may experience discomfort as you are not used to getting so much oxygen and it takes conscious effort to move the diaphragm. Once you practice enough, though, it will become natural, and you will constantly have the benefits of improved blood oxygenation. Deep breathing promotes relaxation, clear thinking, and has rejuvenating effects on your system.

Proper diet and filling your lungs to capacity with each breath are the best means to see that the respiratory component of the body's detoxifying system is working optimally.

THE KIDNEYS

As does the liver, the kidneys act as a blood filtration unit, screening the entire bloodstream, drawing out harmful substances, and discarding them through the urine.

During a detoxification program it is very important to increase water intake, which help the kidneys in their purification job. Drinking three cups of green tea daily and two liters of bottled or filtered water will help flush toxins from the body. Eating plenty of fresh fruits and vegetables and adding chlorophyll or lemon to the drinking water will also stimulate diuresis and help the kidneys cleanse the blood from impurities.

Glancing over the last few pages, we can see that a detoxification program really has two major goals. One is to exhaustively clean out any residual toxins, from excess mucus in the lungs to damaging microbes in the intestines, that have escaped expulsion by the normal operation of the immune system. The other is to "set the house in order," that is, make sure all the interlinked detoxifying organs and systems in the body are functioning at peak levels. These two goals are counterpoints. When the body is overstuffed with toxins, the detoxifying systems cannot work up to snuff because they are overtaxed. When the body is free of excessive toxins, then, as long as healthy living continues, the detoxifiers will keep any buildup from recurring.

De-acidification

The human body functions within certain narrow parameters. Some of these are well-known, such as comfortable temperature ranges; while others, such as pH level, are not widely discussed.

PH level refers simply to the balance between acids and alkalis (or bases) in the body's fluids. Acids and alkalis are complementary chemical compounds that form the basis of many molecular reactions, and which, when combined, form a salt. The chemistry involved may not seem very relevant, but remember that the body works through a mesh of finely calibrated chemical and electrical reactions and needs a specific internal environment to carry out these reactions with full vigor.

For the body to function normally, blood pH must range between 7.35 and 7.45. These numbers indicate a slightly alkaline state. Any value below 7.0 is considered acidic, any value above 7.0 is alkaline.

In the body there are complex biochemical processes called buffering systems that work to keep the blood pH within this narrow range. This function is critical, as even slight deviations from normal pH have a profound impact on all metabolic functions. A shift in pH range will result in decreased oxygen delivery to cells, impaired mineral balance, altered enzymatic-metabolic function, and an increased tendency to develop infectious and chronic-degenerative diseases. In fact, checking the blood and saliva pH is one of the first things to do if one is experiencing illness.

While detoxification aims to remove the presence of bacteria or other germ types that either cause disease directly or interfere with healthy cell operation, deacidification, which should accompany detoxification, is set on making sure blood pH is at a proper level. If it is not, then the very pathogens and toxins that were driven out by detoxing will reappear since an over-acidic pH will encourage their tenancy once they get back into the body.

This deacidification is particularly crucial to Americans, since we favor a diet filled with acidic substances, from red meats to dairy products to shellfish. These lower the blood pH as do many prescription drugs, coffee, nicotine, and stress. To reverse this pH decline we need to reverse our eating patterns.

NECESSARY DIETARY CHANGES TO OBTAIN PROPER pH

As noted, one should avoid eating or reduce consumption of dairy products, meat, seafood, and coffee. We can add to the list of foods and beverages to steer clear of: most grain products and nuts (except millet and almonds), white sugar, chocolate, soft drinks, alcohol, black tea, processed and refined vegetable oils and fats, and vinegar (except apple cider vinegar). Certain foods, although nonacid-forming on their own, may become so when combined with other foods. Citrus fruits for example, are extremely alkalizing, yet if taken with starches, become acid forming.

What should be eaten in abundance when you are embarked on a course of deacidification are dark green leafy vegetables, avocados, almonds, millet, and fresh fruit. Limes and lemons seem acid, but their effect on the body is alkalizing. When deacidifying, it is useful to eat one to two lemons a day. You can mix lemon with orange or grapefruit juice, squeeze it in drinking water, or use it as condiment for veggies and salads. And if you have a lemon, you can make lemonade.

You might want to try this tangy lemon thirst quencher.

SPICY LEMONADE

In a blender mix:

       juice of 2 lemons
       1 carrot
       1 tablespoon flax seed oil
       1 tablespoon maple syrup or raw honey

1/2 cup of pure water
pinch of cayenne pepper
pinch of sea salt

By following this dietary advice, a shift in the body's pH toward alkalinity can be achieved. With the blood so ordered, it will bathe the body with a fluid that is salubrious for healthy bacteria and cells, but inimical to invasive microorganism.

This alone, though, won't optimize the internal environment, for that one also needs the proper mental state, that of stoical calm and life-affirming joy.

De-stressing

We all have had the experience of coming down with a cold or flu in periods of increased tension. The mind and body are inextricably intertwined. Negative thoughts set up a cascade of biochemical responses that inversely affect the functioning of our cells, weakening our immunity, and making us more susceptible to diseases. In addition, stress increases oxidative status, creating free radicals, which are high-energy molecules that damage cells and are involved in degenerative diseases as well as aging. Stress also increases adrenaline production, which itself encourages free radical production.

A number of valuable de-stressing techniques, such as tai chi, can only be understood with some knowledge of the general life philosophies they embody, so they will be covered in section seven at which point their general treatment strategies, world views, and de-stressing techniques can be viewed in integrated form. For now, we will confine our remarks to comments on meditation, a primary means of setting the mind at rest and establishing humane priorities. We want to say something about not only the inner peace meditation affords, but the kind of changes a person who takes meditation seriously is likely to make.

There are many different ways to meditate and re-connect to our inner quietness. Dr. Herbert Benson in his book *The Relaxation Response* "has documented the uniquely altered quality of the meditative state; not like sleeping but not like being fully awake."[10] Benson shows that this meditiave state has a unique profile in metabolism, breathing pace, heartbeat, and other physical parameters. Where stress elevates all these levels, meditation dims them down to a more quiescent form, which resembles sleep except that one remains conscious.

Author Mark Harris calls our attention to the paradox of meditation. "On the surface the most solitary of acts, meditation can break through that sense of individual isolation or loneliness...so common to modern life."[11]

Ultimately, there is no greater purpose in life than realizing who we really are. Yet, this brings us to a second paradox: Our deepest self is not a striving ego, but almost a disembodied presence that is both part of the self and part of others. As awareness of this increases, we naturally start adhering to the values and principles that honor life in everyone. (In the conclusion, we will analyze this paradox as explained by philosopher G. H. Mead.)

Harris lays out the basics of meditation. Once you find a place where you won't be disturbed, sit down in a comfortable position and choose a word or phrase that has a deep meaning. Close your eyes and repeat the word or phrase. Try to keep your attention on nothing but this "mantra," and redirect your mind to it if you drift off into irrelevant thoughts. Do this for ten to twenty minutes. When coming out of meditation, do so slowly. Remain seated for another minute as the concerns of the mundane flow back.

Let's add here that as your concern for others enriches, you will feel you need support, so as to share long-suppressed feelings, reinforce intuition, and build stamina to overcome everyday conditionings and the power of habits. This is something we will take up more forcefully in the conclusion, but for now we can recommend you take time to find a support group where your aspirations and values are cultivated and nurtured, where your questions are answered, and your doubts are welcomed.

And remember: real transformation will occur only if accompanied by changes in lifestyle. This is why it is so important to learn a new way of eating, to rediscover your body through physical exercise, to eliminate the toxins you have accumulated through the years, and regain vitality and clarity of thinking.

Meditation, which induces a tranquillity that allows one to view his or her life without regret, recrimination or inflated pride, feeds back into an unthreatened desire to live in a way that will harmonize with the rediscovered inner quiet. Such a life is one where the natural health of the body is allowed full flower, stoked by exercise, proper diet, and other practices. It will also be satisfied by supplementing the diet with an intake of immune-boosting herbs, minerals, and vitamins.

Immune-Boosting Herbs

All the techniques presented in the previous paragraphs are geared to enhance your immunity. Proper diet, exercise, and avoidance of drinking, smoking, and environmental toxins including unnecessary prescription and over-the-counter drugs, strongly impact our immunity. Maintenance of an alkaline inner environment optimizes the function of our defense mechanisms and creates an unfavorable habitat for the growth of foreign microorganisms. Reducing the amount of mental, emotional, and physical stress will free the immune system from the inhibitory effects of hormones and neuromediators that are released into the bloodstream in response to distress.

In addition to these changes, we can supplement our diets with herbs and nutrients that nourish, support, and enhance the activity of the immune system. Some of these herbs and nutrients also exert direct antimicrobial activity and are precious tools in the fight against infections.

As mentioned at the beginning of this third part, besides possessing these positive qualities, another selling point of herbs and nutrients is that they generally lack the drawbacks of strong side effects that we associate with pharmaceutical products. Antibiotics, for example, when overused may cause selection of resistant and more aggressive bacteria, side effects and allergic reactions. Moreover, these conventional drugs can suppress the activity of the immune system and increase the likelihood of recurrent infections. Recent research for example, has shown that children treated with antibiotics for respiratory infections were much more likely to develop subsequent recurrent infections than untreated children.[12]

CAUTIONS CONCERNING HERB USE

Let's restrict ourselves to herbs for a moment. At this point, the reader probably expects me to extol herbs as being faultless in respect to side effects. However, rather than follow that path, let me do the unexpected and admit that herbs have been known to have negative side effects, although herb bashers tend to magnify or write unclearly about what is wrong.

For instance, an April 2000 issue of medical magazine *AORN Journal* bannered "Consuming Chinese Herbs May Cause Kidney Failure." Granted that a new study did show twelve patients taking herbs had kidney failure, and thus these herbs are problematic. However, reading further, one finds they were not simply taking particular herbs, but a herbal "slimming" formula. Such packets may contain things other than herbs. Besides, which herbs as well as what other natural pharmaceuticals might have been in the packet were not specified. Indeed, the Taiwan researchers said "no common ingredient was identified."[13]

Another instance of unclear indictments of herbs is noted by Rob McCaleb of the Herb Research Foundation. He mentions that when *JAMA* (the *Journal of the American Medical Association*) takes time to assail the use of herbs, it is not necessarily done on the firmest foundation. McCaleb cites an article from *JAMA*'s July 11, 2000, issue, which says problems can arise for surgical patients who supplement with gingko, St. John's wort, garlic, ginseng, or other herbs. However, a close reading of the *JAMA* piece shows the disparaging of various herbs is based either on no (in the case of echinacea) or flawed evidence. For the danger of garlic supplements, for example, the only case used to point to the dangers of pre-surgery patients using this supplement, "did not even involve the use of a garlic supplement, but a rather extreme consumption of the food. One elderly man ate...about five medium-sized garlic cloves a day for an extended period."[14]

Nonetheless, for all its bumbling, the *JAMA* article is putting its finger on a danger that can arise with herb consumption, which is that adverse reactions may occur when they are taken during the time one is undergoing conventional medical procedures or taking traditional drugs. "Toxic interactions can occur between herbs and existing medications or therapies."[15] Bear in mind, the same thing can happen when two conventional meds are mixed or when conventional drugs are taken in conjunction with certain foods. A particular difficulty is that patients who try to combine traditional and alternative therapies, may be bouncing between two practitioners without informing either of the existence of the other.

> Patients who consume herbs seldom disclose this information to their physicians or other [conventional] health care providers. Whether they believe they are stigmatized or just believe herbs are equivalent to vitamins and thus relatively harmless, many fail to realize an herb's potential for medication...interaction [with traditional drugs].[16]

When you see a health practitioner, full disclosure of what treatments and medications, herbs, and nutrients you are currently using is necessary. Any other course will lead to trouble.

However, we are not mentioning the danger of drug/herb interactions as a way of sidestepping the main theme. Many herbs do have side effects. An article in the *Townsend Letter for Doctors and Patients* highlights, among a number of examples, that garlic can lower thyroid function, which can be disastrous for patient with weak thyroid action.[17] Rather than go further in enumerating side effects at this moment, I will mention any adverse reactions that are tied to a particular immune-boosting herb when I cover that herb in the listing that follows.

And remember, even if we acknowledge that some herbs have been shown to be associated with troubling consequence, the earlier point still holds. Herbs do not cause anywhere near the panoply of problems we find with prescription drugs. As Dr. James A. Duke writes, "Prescription drugs are killing 140,000 Americans a year. Herbs (usually through abuse or exceeding recommended dosage) are killing fewer than one hundred."[18] Herb-bashers, such as the *JAMA* author, might counter that many more people take physicians' prescription drugs than take herbs, although the real numbers of the second group would be difficult to ascertain, since, as we saw, many users are reluctant to admit they take the natural medicines. However, given the comparative death rates, one questions the priorities of those who publicly worry about health hazards of herbs but say nothing about the menace of prescribed medications.

It is also worth mentioning that aside from side effects, two other problems those who use herbs should be aware of are a possible lack of freshness and the dangers of standardization.

Recently, there has been a trend to standardize bottled herbs. This means the percentage of the plant's active compounds in each dose are guaranteed on the label. However, some, such as Dr. Duke, argue that such standardization takes us away from the essence of plant remedies. "Plants are just as variable as people," he says. "We should not expect individual plants to be any more alike than you and me."[19]

Nonetheless, many would say Duke is off track, since if one doesn't know one is getting a good potency of active elements in a herb, taking it may be wasted effort. However, this is based on the assumption that herbalists have correctly identified the major active components. Since herbs contain hundreds of compounds, the label will only mention those that are considered key to the herb's healing actions. However, as Jack Challem, writing in *Natural Health*, notes, there is a danger that ingredients will be mistakenly given powers they don't have. He mentions, along with other example, that of hypercin, which was long considered the key antidepressant factor in St. John's wort, and was duly standardized. "However, a couple of years ago, researchers discovered that hypercin has antiviral not antidepressant properties."[20] In other cases, a compound listed as key may turn out not to be essential after all.

Moreover, even if an ingredient has been correctly assessed, there is still the possibility that it alone is not responsible for the ultimate benefits the herb provides. A single herb contains hundreds of chemicals, Duke reminds us. "Herbs...possess a great variety of biologically active compounds, which evolved to defend and support the herb, often in synergy."[21] From his viewpoint, an herb's phytochemicals work in an integrated fashion, and the thought that any one compound is the prime mover is erroneous.

None of this carping knocks out the value of the herbals, it only undercuts the value of standardization.

Of course, most herbalist would say the best way to imbibe herbs is to get them fresh. And for those of us who live in cities and don't have access to fresh herbs, second best is getting them in dried form. However, dried herbs that have been sitting in a store too long will have lost their potency, so it is important to be careful in selecting ones to purchase. Judy Krizmanic provides advice on what to watch for in picking out herbs. Some of the most significant recommendations she has are to examine the color of the herbs, smell them, and try to get them as whole as possible. Here are the details:

> Dried herbs should resemble the color they were when fresh.... [When trying to gauge the quality offered in a

particular store] find a dried herb that you know is bright green while it grows, such as mint, and look for a dried version that retains a similar hue.

You want to find herbs that have a distinctive strong aroma.... Check out the culinary herbs you are familiar with, such as basil or thyme, and use them as a test of the store's general quality.

Whole roots and leaves provide a natural package for a plant's delicate medicucinal [medical and culinary] constituents. Ground and powdered herbs are much more volatile.... See if your store's herb buyer can get [whole roots and leaves].[22]

Now that we have seen that herbs, like anything we consume, need to be chosen with circumspection and thoughtful consideration, let's look at some herbs with proven immune-boosting power, which can be made part of your health enhancing program.

Herb Lexicon

ARTICHOKE LEAVES *(Cynara scolymus)*

Artichoke leaves protect the liver from damage and help effectuate its detoxifying powers. This has been the subject of study for the last seventy years. In one study, for instance, done in the 1950s, "researchers gave extract of artichoke leaves to dozens of Polish workers who had been exposed to fumes from carbon disulfide, a potent liver toxin. The workers did not experience any of the liver damage that the toxin typically causes."[23]

Eating whole artichokes will give you all the medicinal dose you need of the plant, but keep in mind that the heart, which many find the most scrumptious part of the vegetable, has less potency than the leaves.

ASHWAGANDHA *(Withania somnifera)*

Also called Indian ginseng, in India ashwagandha is used as a general tonic especially for men, due to its anti-aging properties. Studies have shown that ashwagandha possesses anti-inflammatory, anti-stress, antioxidant, and immunomodulatory properties.[24] The effects on the immune system are multiple, increasing the number and the activity of white blood cells, enhancing antibody production, and increasing macrophage function.[25]

The dried root can be taken in tincture (2–4 ml three times per day), in capsules (3–6 grams) or as a tea. (ml = milliliter.) For the tea, use two teaspoons of root per cup of water, boiled for fifteen minutes. It can be taken three times per day.

ASTRAGALUS (*Astragalus membranaceus*)

Astragalus is native to China, where it is known as *huang qi*, "yellow leader," which refers to the color of the root and its role in Chinese traditional medicine as one of the most important tonic herbs. It can be safely taken for long periods of time to boost the immune system, prevent illnesses, and assist the body in recovering from infections and long-term chronic conditions.

Herb manuals refer to it as an adaptogen. Adaptogens are herbs that help the body face stress assault. In other words, when you are put into a high-anxiety situation, in work, at home or in any circumstances, these herbs are said to help your body to adapt to this new level of strain, so that it can move through the pressure without weakening of the health or of mental outlook.

Astragalus also has a powerful antiviral activity, derived from its ability to increase the activity of natural killer cells and stimulate the production of alpha- and gamma-interferon, important parts of the body's response to viral infection. In addition astragalus enhances macrophage activity, increases the number of circulating white blood cells, stimulates their maturation into active cells, and increases antibody production. This herb is an all-around immune system aid.

Astragalus can be taken in capsules (three capsules three times per day) or tincture (3–5 ml three times per day). The root can be used to make a decoction or added to soups. To make a decoction boil the root in water for a few minutes and then brew the tea.

BARBERRY (*Berberis vulgaris*)

Barberry is native to Europe, but grows throughout North America. It contains berberine, the antibiotic compound also present in goldenseal. Besides being antibiotic, this herb has anti-bacterial and anti-parasitic properties. It works by preventing microbes from attaching to human cells, rather than by directly killing the intruders.

Barberry can be taken in tincture (2–4 ml three times per day), capsules (3–20 capsules per day), ointment for topical applications, and as a tea (use 1 heaping teaspoon per cup of boiling water).

BEARBERRY (*Arctostaphlos uva-ursi*)

Bearberry is an evergreen found throughout Europe and in North America and Britain. It has proven particularly useful, due to its antimicrobial properties, in helping with kidney problems, as with ulcerations, cystitis, and other chronic diseases. As we've seen, the kidney is one of the cleansing organs of the body, and it needs to be in peak working order to maintain internal detoxification.

As an infusion, bearberry should be taken three times a day. Preparation involves pouring a cup of hot water on two teaspoons of the dried leaves, letting the cup sit for fifteen minutes. As a tincture, take 2–3 ml three times a day.

ECHINACEA
(*Echinacea purpurea, Echinacea angustifolia, Echinacea pallida*)

Echinacea bolsters the immune system and helps the body fight infection. The plant is native to North America, where three main species exist: *E. purpurea, E. angustifolia, E. pallida.*

Echinacea is effective against a broad range of bacteria, viruses, fungi, and protozoa. The herb increases the number and the activity of all the white blood cells (including lymphocytes, macrophages, neutrophils, and natural killers), and stimulates production of interferon.

It also has a special task in defending the integrity of our ialuronic acid. Our tissues contain ialuronic acid, a molecule that builds a protective wall against pathogens. Many such pathogens produce an enzyme, called hyaluronidase, which dissolves molecules of ialuronic acid, creating a port of entry for the invaders. Studies have shown that echinacea prevents the activity of this hole-creating enzyme, therefore denying germs access to the body's cells.

In addition to increasing the body's ability to fight off infections, echinacea possesses direct antiviral activity. One studied showed that cultured cells grown in a medium containing echinacea were more resistant to influenza and herpes viruses. According to Janet Zand, OMD, echinacea proven action against the flu is based on how the herb "increases the number of phagocytes in the blood."[26]

Echinacea can be taken in tincture, capsules or decoctions. During an infection, 3–4 ml of tincture should be taken every two hours, the dosage being gradually reduced as symptoms improve. Tinctures usually are stronger than capsules and work faster, being more easily absorbed into the bloodstream. As an alternative, two to three capsules three times per day may be taken. To make a decoction, add two teaspoons of root per cup of water, bring to a boil, and simmer for fifteen minutes. Drink three to four cups per day. In capsule form, Zand recommends taking two (of 500–1000 mg) on the same tapering off schedule used with tinctures.

It is probably best to use a blend of all types of echinacea, as they have been shown to work well together. In addition, combining echinacea with other herbs, such as goldenseal and astragalus, will greatly enhance its activity

ELDERBERRY (*Sambucus nigra*)

Elderberry grows as a common shrub in Europe and North America. Both the flowers and the berries are used medicinally.

The herb contains compounds that are active against influenza, Epstein-Barr and herpes simplex viruses. Its anti-influenza activity was shown, for example, in a double-blind study conducted in Israel. Ninety percent of flu sufferers who used the extract were better in from two to three days, whereas it took at minimum six days to have resolution of symptoms in those who took a placebo. In vitro studies backed up these claims.[27]

The fruit of elderberry is sometimes used to make jellies and jams. This could be a nice way to get your medicine.

Otherwise you can use it as a tincture (use 5 ml in children, 10 ml in adults, twice a day) or make a tea (steeping two teaspoons of dried flowers in a cup of boiling water for ten minutes, and drinking three cups a day).

GARLIC (*Allium sativum*)

The use of garlic to treat infections dates back to the ancient Egyptians, Greeks, and Romans. During World War II, garlic saved thousands of lives in Russia, when it was used to keep wounds from becoming infected when the nation's antibiotic supply was overwhelmed by the high number of casualties.

Research has shown that garlic inhibits the growth of and kills several species of bacteria and fungi, being active against some of the most virulent pathogens, such as the bacteria that causes tuberculosis, and the fungus that causes the often fatal cryptococcal meningitis.[28] Antiviral activity has been documented against selected viruses including, herpes simplex virus cytomegalovirus, vaccinia virus, vesicular stomatitis virus, parainfluenza virus, human rhinovirus, and HIV virus.[29] In relation to strengthening immune function, garlic gets involved...in supporting gastrointestinal action in the way it will support the development of the natural bacterial flora whilst killing pathogenic organisms."[30]

In view of the strong antibiotic properties and the complete absence of development of microbial resistance to the plant, garlic use as broad-spectrum therapeutic agent merits special consideration.

There are several sulfur compounds in garlic that have antimicrobial properties. The key ingredient, allicin, "protects the plant from soil parasites and fungi and is also responsible for garlic's pungent smell."[31] You may notice that this odor is not sensible on a peeled clove, but it will be overwhelmingly in evidence if the clove is crushed. This is because allicin itself is not present in the fresh garlic, but two precursor molecules are, and these come together, producing the key compound, when the clove is squashed. This also tells us that uncompressed garlic should not be eaten as it will be lacking its most potent element. If you consume raw garlic, first crush it with a spoon to release the allicin. When eaten, garlic gets digested and its active ingredients are absorbed into the bloodstream. The herb is excreted via the lungs, hence the strong sulfur-type odor of the breath after eating garlic. This mode of elimination makes it very active against different types of respiratory infections.

Work done at the Weizmann Institute of Science in Israel has given us more understanding of how garlic proceeds against germs. What allicin does is interfere with two groups of enzymes: cysteine proteinases and alcohol dehydrogenases. The first group helps pathogens invade and attack hosts, the second is necessary for the antigens' survival.

> Because these groups of enzymes are found in a wide variety of infectious organisms such as bacteria, fungi, and viruses, this research provides a scientific basis for the notion that allicin…is capable of warding off different types of infections."[32]

Moreover, the protection afforded by allicin would be hard to beat by wily germs, such at those that are adept at switching outer identificatory proteins to disguise themselves, since the enzyme groups targeted by allicin are vital to pathogen metabolism. These enzymes, scientists have concluded, would be hard for pathogens to replace.

Garlic is best eaten raw or taken with foods. Eat one clove three times a day. Some will have trouble tolerating the smell, and some practitioners say enteric-coated capsules with standardized allicin potential can be used in the amount of roughly 1 gram of garlic divided in three daily doses (providing up to 6,000 mcg of allicin potential). Others advise against anything but raw form garlic. Dr. Joseph Mercola writes, "The active ingredient is destroyed within one hour of smashing the garlic. Garlic pills are virtually worthless."[33] Rarely, users of garlic will suffer from gastrointestinal upset, alterations of intestinal flora, and allergic reactions; and so these should be watched for.

GINGER (*Zingiber officinale*)

Ginger was first described in China's herbal, the *Pen Tsao Ching* (*Classic of Herbs*), which dates to approximately 3000 BCE. Since then it has been noted for its ability to help the immune system drive off infectious pathogens, showing particular power against flu and cold viruses.

Ginger root is a pleasure to take since it can be blended in with fruit and vegetables juices, added to soups, vegetarian stew or rice. It can also be made into a tea or swallowed as a capsule. For juices and soups, up to a inch of root can be used, according to personal taste. To make ginger tea, use two teaspoons of grated root per cup of boiling water. Steep this mixture ten minutes. In capsules, two to four grams of ginger may be used daily.

GINSENGS

AMERICAN GINSENG (*Panax quinquefolus*)

This plant with its dark green leaves and red berries grows in the Eastern United States and is a close relative of Korean ginseng. Its effect is milder than but comparable to that of the other ginsengs, and so it can be taken to provide similar immune-strengthening value "without overstimulation to those people with high levels of stress and mental stimulation."[34] It is said to strengthen the lungs to help them fight off pathogen intrusion and to aid in recovery from infectious diseases.

This ginseng can be made into a tea. The root should be cut up and simmered in water for forty-five minutes. The procedure should not be done in a metal pot since this may weaken the plant's antioxidant properties. One can have two or three cups a day. The tea can also be made with ginseng powder or the powder can be swished into juice or water for a cool drink. Use one half to one teaspoon of the powder per glass.

Pregnant women should not take any ginseng. No adverse reactions have been recorded for those who stay within normal dosage, nonetheless, it should not be taken long term but rather when one is sick or is undergoing an immune-strengthening regimen.

ASIAN GINSENG (*Panax ginseng*)

Asian ginseng is another tonic herb, which has been part of Chinese traditional medicine for more than two thousand years.

Let me add, parenthetically, that you will often see such references to the way various herbs have a history dating back to ancient times. The reference is usually to India or China, since these countries have the longest, continuous medical traditions. All this is not said just to impress the reader. The fact is, though many moderns will sneer at older, foreign medical practices, which, indeed, lack the knowledge of disease gained through the nineteenth and twentieth centuries, these older medicines were pragmatic. A herb that didn't get results was dropped out of their *Materia Medica*. Herbs, like ginseng, that stayed the course must have some had some intrinsic fighting, energizing, or supportive ability.

Asian ginseng is used as a general stimulator, primarily for men. It also enhances immune function.

This ginseng contains a wide array of active compounds, including ginsenosides, which increase energy, reduce stress, and enhance physical and mental performance, and polysaccharides with their immune-stimulating ability.

Ginseng can be taken in powdered form (1/4 teaspoon a day) or in capsules. Standardized extract may be taken in the amount of 100–200 mg per day, increasing the dose up to two grams per day for non-standardized extracts. Ginseng is usually taken continuously for three weeks, followed by a one to two week break before resuming. It is best to avoid taking it at night, as it may cause overexcitation and insomnia.

SIBERIAN GINSENG OR ELEUTHERO (*Eleutherococcus senticosus*)

Eleuthero is frequently called Siberian ginseng, although it does not belong to the ginseng family. It has, however, the ginseng-like properties of being an energizer and immune enhancer. It is much used in the former Soviet Union, and was given by Russian authorities to its citizens to counteract the mutagenicity of radiations after the Chernobyl accident.

Among its active constituents are eleutherosides, molecules that have been shown to enhance immune system function in test-tube and animal experiments. Other compounds have shown antioxidant, anticancer, antibacterial, and glucose- and cholesterol-lowering activity.[35]

Eleuthero can be taken in tincture or capsules. Two to three grams of powdered root can be used daily, or 400 mg of extract standardized for its eleutheroside content. Generally, it is taken over a six to eight week period, followed by a two-week break before resuming intake.

"The side effects of ginseng typically are mild and dose related. The most commonly observed side effects are nervousness, sleeplessness, skin eruptions,...leg and ankle swelling, dizziness, and diarrhea."[36] Anyone suffering these adverse reactions should discontinue use.

GOLDENSEAL (*Hydrastis canadensis*)

Goldenseal is a herb native to eastern North America, used by the Native Americans for skin wounds and eye infections, respiratory tract infections, and gastroenteritis. Today the herb is close to extinction because of over-harvesting in the wild; so, when possible, other herbs with similar activity, such as barberry or Oregon grape, should be used.

Goldenseal contains two active compounds, berberine and hydrastine. Berberine, an alkaloid compound also present in barberry and Oregon grape, has wide-spectrum antimicrobial activity against germs that cause diarrhea, such as *E. coli*, *Salmonella typhi*, and *Entamoeba histolytica*.

Goldenseal is also a mild immune stimulant, enhancing the activity of macrophages, but its main action remains that of killing bacteria and parasites.

Goldenseal can be taken as an infusion, but it has a very bitter taste. Add one teaspoon of powdered root to a cup of boiling water. Steep for ten minutes. Sweeten with maple syrup or honey to improve the flavor and drink two to three cups per day.

For tinctures, 2–4 ml three times per day are used. For capsules, doses vary with standardized (500 mg three times per day) and non-standardized extracts (2 grams three times per day). Dosages may be increased to up to twenty-five capsules a day in cases of more severe infections; but these higher dosages should be administered under the supervision of a qualified health professional as gastrointestinal side effects may develop.

Goldenseal, unlike most of the immune stimulants discussed in this section, is not known as a preventative. It is effective in treating infections, and intake should be suspended at resolution of symptoms when taken for this purpose. However, some practitioners, such as Janet Zand, OMD, see that a reduced dosage can be used to prime the body for infection assault. Zand writes, "For prevention...a combination of echinacea and Goldenseal may be taken two or three times daily for one to two weeks per month." She finds this is useful "during the cold, hayfever and allergy season when the body is often under stress."[37]

GREEN TEA (*Camellia sinensis*)

Green tea, black tea, and white tea all derive from the same plant, *Camellia sinensis*. What differs is how the leaves are prepared. Black tea, for example, is obtained through fermentation; while green tea leaves are only lightly steamed. Green tea, which goes through less processing, keeps the plant's active constituents, particularly polyphenols, effective.

In traditional Chinese medicine green tea is used to increase energy levels and enhance the activity of the immune system. Test tube and animal studies have given us a better idea of how this enhancement operates. The green tea builds up humoral and cell-mediated immunity (both sides of the system), increasing the number and activity of B and T lymphocytes, and of natural killer cells. In addition, the extract modifies the intestinal microflora, reducing undesirable bacteria and increasing beneficial bacteria. This effect could make it a valuable supplement to re-equilibrate gut flora during antibiotic therapy.

Green tea extract has demonstrated antimicrobial and microbicidal activity against a wide spectrum of pathogens, such as *staphylococci* and *Yersinia enterocolitica, Vibrio cholerae, Salmonella typhimurium* and *Salmonella typhi, Mycoplasma pneumoniae*, Shigella, *V. parahaemolyticus*, and *enteropathogenic E. coli*.[38] The bactericidal activity often occurred at the drinking concentration in daily life. In addition, green tea catechins can inhibit the release of Vero toxin from enterohemorrhagic *Escherichia coli* O157:H7, the strain of *E. coli* that was used during the bioterrorism attack in Oregon.[39]

What is even more interesting is that green tea extract is capable of killing even some antibiotic resistant germs, such as methicillin-resistant *Staphylococcus aureus* and, to some extent, penicillin-resistant *S. aureus*.[40] One of the mechanisms by which bacteria develop antibiotic resistance is through spontaneous mutation accompanied by selective pressure of antibiotics given at sub-optimal doses. Cathechins can inhibit spontaneous mutations in bacteria at doses well below those required to induce direct bactericidal action. These effects are exerted against resistance to tetracyclines, fluoroquinolones, macrolides, beta-lactams, and aminoglycosides, and could have important impact in practical antibiotic therapy.[41]

Green tea can be taken as a beverage or in capsules. To achieve the health benefits documented in populations consuming green tea regularly, drink at least three cups of tea daily, prepared with one heaping teaspoon of tea per cup of water. Be sure to purchase good quality tea, with a high content of polyphenols. Capsules containing extracts standardized for 80 percent total polyphenol are also available, a daily dose of 400 mg being equivalent to three cups of tea.

LIGUSTRUM (*Ligustrum lucidum*)

Ligustrum is often used in traditional Chinese medicine in combination with astragalus to stimulate the immune system. Several studies have proved its ability to enhance and modulate immune function, inhibit tumor growth, and protect the liver from toxicity.[42]

Ligustrum can be imbibed in tinctures (2–4 ml, three times per day) or capsules (3–10 grams per day), or can be taken as tea. For the beverage, add one to two teaspoons of powdered berries to a cup of boiling water and steep for ten minutes. It is a safe herb, and no common side effects have been described.

MILK THISTLE (*Silybum marinum*)

This prickly weed is grown throughout much of the world and is known for protecting the liver, allowing it to proceed with its cleaning function efficiently. Since the liver is under constant siege in our contemporary world from environmental toxins, secondary smoke, food additives, and pollutants, supporting it with all means possible is important.

Milk thistle dramatically proved its worth in the 1970s when "one researcher gave silymarin [the active ingredient in milk thistle] to sixty people who had developed severe liver poisoning from accidentally eating wild Amanitat mushrooms." On average, 30 to 40 percent of those who ingest these mushrooms die, but with the silymarin "every single subject survived."[43]

A standard recommended dose is 70–210 mg, three times a day, in capsule form. You can also buy milk thistle seeds and grind them up to sprinkle on cooked grains. They are slightly bitter, however, and some may not like them for eating for this reason.[44]

MYRRH (*Commiphora myrrha*)

Myrrh, well known to many due its mention as an oil in the Bible, is the gum resin of a Northern African plant. It stimulates the production of white blood cells, the building blocks of the immune system, as well as attacks invading microbes on its own. Studies have shown myrrh to be particularly effective against infections of the mouth, such as gingivitis and mouth ulcers, and for throat infections, such as laryngitis.

As a tincture, one should take 1–4 ml three times a day. Although this is a less convenient way to obtain it, it can also be swallowed as an infusion. To make this, pour a cup of boiling water onto one to two teaspoons of powdered myrrh and let it infuse for ten to fifteen minutes. Drink this three times a day.[45]

MUSHROOMS

Maitake, shiitake, and reishi mushroom have been used for thousands of years to increase energy and boost immunity. Research is now confirming their antiviral and immunostimulant properties.

MAITAKE *(Grifola frondosa)*

The maitake mushroom is found in Japan. The word "mai" in Japanese means dance and so, as medical researcher Mark Mayell notes, this means the maitake is "the dancing mushroom." Perhaps it got this name because "the fruiting bodies of adjacent fungi overlap each other, looking like nymphs or butterflies in a wild dance."[46]

All medicinal mushrooms have complex polysaccharides in their structure, which account for their immuno-modulating properties. Maitake's primary polysaccharide, beta D-glucan, has shown particular promise as an adjunct to cancer and HIV therapy, because of its immune system–potentiating powers.

It was the research done in the 1980s by Dr. Hiroaki Nanba at the Pharmaceutical University of Kobe that laid the basis for an understanding of maitake's medicinal properties. Nanba discovered a fraction (component) of the mushroom that had the ability to stimulate macrophages. Other studies have shown that maitake can be used to prevent or treat liver disease. "Chinese researchers conducted a pilot study on thirty-two patients with chronic hepatitis B...those patients who took a maitake fruit body polysaccharide preparation showed positive signs," as against those who took standard treatment.[47]

Maitake can be taken as food (remember that the fruit body has higher polysaccharide content than the mycelium), or in capsules (4–8 grams per day can be used). Liquid preparations high in polysaccharide concentrations are also available.

SHITAKE (*Lentinus edodes*)

This tasty Asian mushroom has been prized for thousands of years in China and Japan as food and medicinal herb. Research has shown that shitake contains a polysaccharide, called lentinan, with impressive immunostimulant, antiviral, and antitumor effects. Shitake has been shown to inhibit replication of herpes simplex and HIV virus.[48] Shitake mobilizes the immune system by increasing the number and the activity of lymphocytes, and stimulates production of interferon. Although the mechanism of its antitumor action is still not completely clear, it is suggested that its polysaccharides activate the host defense system through stimulation of many kinds of immune cells, T-lymphocytes, macrophages, natural killer cells, and induction of various immunomodulatory molecules with anti-viral and anti-tumor properties, which are essential to maintain homeostasis.[49]

Shitake can be taken in powder or capsules, or you can use the whole mushroom as food, over salads or in soups. An extract of the mycelium, called LEM (*lentinus edodes mycelium* extract), prepared from the mycelium before the cap and stem are grown, is rich in active substances and is more potent than the crude mushroom. Take 2–3 grams three times a day.

REISHI (*Ganoderma lucidum*)

Reishi mushrooms are another mainstay of the ancient Chinese pharmacopoeia, having been singled out in that tradition as increasers of vitality and promoters of long life.

Research has shown that reishi possesses immuno-modulant, anti-cancer and antiviral activity.[50] Polysaccharides from fresh fruiting bodies of reishi mushroom stimulate production of molecules with antiviral and anti-cancer activity, such as interleukin-1, tumor necrosis factor, interferon gamma, and interleukin 6. Inhibition of replication of herpes, influenza, and HIV viruses and of the growth of different cancer cell lines has been documented in both in vitro and in vivo experiments.

Reishi can be taken as crude dried mushroom, in capsules (2–4 grams per day), tincture (2–4 ml per day), or as a tea.

OLIVE LEAF EXTRACT

Olives don't only have a place as garnishes to alcoholic beverages. They should also be in the medicine cabinet.

The olive tree is native to the Mediterranean region, southern Russia, and the Middle East, though it has been transplanted to and thrives in South America, Australia, and California. It can reach up to thirty feet in height and is an evergreen.

The leaves of the tree have proven potent against microbes, but most attention has been given to the plant's active ingredient, oleuropein, which is "the stuff that helps protect the tree against insect and bacterial predators."[51] Further pharmaceutical work managed to isolate the most potent chemical agent within oleuropein, which turned out to be elenoic acid.

In the late 1960s, research by scientists at a major American pharmaceutical company showed that elenoic acid...inhibited the growth of viruses. In fact, it stopped every virus that it was tested against.[52]

These students of the viral inhibition phenomenon felt that elenoic acid was making a many-pronged attack by interfering with viruses' production of amino acids and cell membrane and blocking viral replication. Unlike the body's own immune system cells, elenoic acid was able to go into cells the viruses had invaded and make an onslaught against the pathogens from there. At the same time as it goes to bat against antigens, it also stirs up the immune system by boosting the action of phagocytes.

Since that time elenoic acid has been used to treat varied conditions from rheumatoid arthritis to flu, to herpes to bacterial infections. More research has to be done to illuminate what value olive leaf extract has, but, as James R. Privitera, MD, says, "I think we are just beginning to scratch the surface for what seems to be a very promising and unique herbal."[53]

Recommended dosage of olive leaf extract capsules is one 500-mg capsule every six hours, although for acute infection some take up to three capsules four times a day. The extract should not be taken at the same time as antibiotics, amino acids, or any mold or fungus derivatives, because it will cancel out their effect.

OREGON GRAPE (*Berberis aquifolium*)

Oregon grape, a close relative of barberry, and is native to North America. It contains the alkaloid berberine, which accounts for its antimicrobial activity. In vitro studies have demonstrated that Oregon grape can activate macrophage activity.

Oregon grape can be taken in the form of tea by boiling one heaping teaspoon of chopped root in a cup of water for ten minutes. It can also be used as a tincture (2–4 ml three times per day) or taken in capsule form (up to twenty capsules per day). Less is required for standardized extracts.

RODIOLO ROSA

The use of this plant, which grows in the high altitudes in the mountains and Arctic areas of Europe and Asia, illustrates the parochialism of American medicine. As might be guessed, this plant's medicinal benefits have been most studied in countries where it grows wild, particularly in Sweden and Russia. Research into its qualities has continued for thirty-five years, but most of what has been found out is unknown in America because the scientific work has not been translated.

We do know, though, that rodiolo rosa is useful in reducing the disruption that occurs in the immune system at the onset of stress. As an adaptogenic herb, it provides "the ability to be exposed to a stressor, while responding with either decreased or no characteristic hormonal perturbations." Moreover, use of this herb "also implies being prepared to and capable of rapidly reassuming homeostasis after the stressor is withdrawn."[54] Specifically, in animal studies, rodiola has been found to decrease the production of the beta endorphins that are produced under stress. The more of these produced, the less able the body is to ride through stress at an even keel.

If you take this herb, you will be getting in on the ground floor level, since it is not widely known. Human experiments with, for example, students about to take an anxiety-producing test, have found good effects taking about 100 mg a day. At double this dose, side effects have been occasionally seen after a few days' use. The effects are irritability and insomnia. If these appear, dosage should be immediately stopped.

SCHISANDRA

Schisandra is a woody vine found in northern China, Russia, and Korea. It can grow to twenty-five feet in height and has lovely pink flowers. As Belinda Rowland describes it, "Schisandra fruit…appears as numerous spikes of tiny, bright red berries. The berries have sweet, sour, hot, salty, and bitter tastes— hence the Chinese name for Schisandra, *wu wei zi* (five-flavored herb)."[55]

For immune-strengthening, schisandra is important in aiding liver function, being particularly beneficial to those suffering from viral hepatitis. Its helpfulness in this area is due to its possession of lignans. These are chemicals that protect the liver from pathogens and regenerate damaged liver tissue.

Daily dose of the herb should be 1.5 to 15 grams of the dried fruit a day or 2–4 ml of tincture three times a day. It can also be consumed as a powder, 1.5 to 6 grams per day or as a capsule of 1.5 g each day. As a tea, it can be prepared by steeping 1–6 grams of dried berries in one to three cups of boiled water.

It should not be taken by pregnant women or by anyone who has trouble urinating. Occasionally, taking the herb will cause skin rashes, heartburn, upset stomach, and lessened appetite.

WILD INDIGO

This root is collected in the fall after the plant has flowered. It is protective of the lymphatic system and also helps with infections of the mouth. Taken "as a mouthwash it will heal mouth ulcers [and] gingivitis."[56]

As a decoction, it is made by placing one teaspoonful of the herb in a cup of water. The water is boiled then let sit for ten to fifteen minutes. The beverage should be drunken three times a day. If a tincture it preferred, 1–2 ml can be taken three times a day.

Herbal Support for Stress

One problem with the threat of terrorist biological attack and of newly surfacing super germs will be with us whether these attacks or germs appear or not. That is the presence of widespread anxiety as people anticipate the worst.

A January 2002 article in *Amednews* by Victoria Stagg Elliott speaks of the psychological toll of the World Trade Center assault:

> The disaster combined with the anthrax scare...has led physicians to report that they are seeing more depression, anxiety and insomnia among their patients. Patients who are already struggling with mental health issues appear to be getting worse.[57]

The hardest hit areas are Washington, D.C., and environs; New York; and Pennsylvania; but people across the United States have been put into a dark mood. A study by Isis Research, a market research firm that tracks pharmaceutical issues, has seen 43 percent of doctors surveyed are prescribing more antidepressants since the September 11 incident. At the same time, there has been a burgeoning need for more drug and alcohol counseling. Mohammad Kahn, MD, a radiologist from Ann Arbor noted, "This is one of the most underestimated impacts, medically, of a disaster.... There's a critical need for help after a disaster, but there's [also] a real need for it years out."[58]

Bearing this in mind, I want to speak for a moment about herbs that have been known to calm and reduce nervousness. More will be said about the alleviation of tension in our section on alternative therapies.

Dr. Ali, whose comments on water in the diet we already heard, made the following recommendations for herbs that can combat stress.

VALERIAN ROOT will soothe one to sleep in doses of 400 to 1,000 milligrams right before lying down. For those who are suffering especially strong anxiety or sadness, he advises taking 400 to 500 mg three times a day.

CHAMOMILE is useful whether in tea or a capsule of 250 to 400 mg once or twice daily.

ST. JOHN's wort and ginkgo biloba can be taken two or three times a day in dosage ranging from 250 to 500 ml.

PASSION FLOWER, catnip and skullcap, as mild herbs, can be taken in rotation with the above.

Ali reminds herbal users, "First and foremost, it is important to use herbs in moderate doses and in rotation. All herbs become drugs if used in large doses and for long periods of time."[59]

Vitamins, Minerals, and Other Immune-Boosting Nutrients

A long with herbs, nutrients, vitamins, minerals, and trace elements support and re-balance the body's functions, and when used at high doses, they can exert a direct role in suppressing infection.

Their role in preventing and treating illnesses is becoming more important, as we are increasingly exposed to toxins derived from the environment and the food we eat, laced with hundreds of different types of additives and pesticides. In addition, in our society, nutrients deficiencies are extremely common in spite of excessive food intake, because the soil where fruits and vegetables are grown is depleted of vital nutrients. This is why it is very important to buy products grown on organic farms, farms that give time to the soil to replenish itself between crops, where crops are rotated and the soil enriched with vital nutrients, and where toxic chemical fertilizers, pesticides, and herbicides are banned.

The nutrients presented in this chapter are designed to make an individual stronger and more apt to resist, fight, and win the battle against a wide range of diseases. This approach, which can be used alone or in combination with conventional treatments, is designed to make an individual less vulnerable to diseases from the start, maximizing the efficiency of the immune system, and bringing it to its fullest defensive potential against foreign invaders.

BEE PRODUCTS

BEE POLLEN

Pollen is a yellowish grain produced by plants for reproductive purposes. When bees fly from flower to flower to collect this pollen for their own use, they moisten it with honey brought from the hive, rolling it into a ball with all the pollen collected from other flowers. "In the course of her work, a pollen forager [bee] will visit as many as 1,500 blossoms."[60]

Bee pollen is chock full of vitamins, minerals, amino acids, and protein. It can be obtained as a harvested substance or mixed in with unprocessed honey. Most honey sold in supermarkets lacks this beneficial additive. "Honey in supermarkets...[is] a refined liquid sweet with all the bits of pollen and propolis strained out. Unfortunately, only a true unrefined raw honey can be classified as a nutritive food."[61]

It should be cautioned that some people are allergic to this and other bee-created substances and so should test their allergic reaction to such products before taking them. However, bee pollen itself has been found to reduce hay fever and other flower pollen-based allergies. To put this in another way, bee pollen helps modulate the immune system's reactions so that it does not make an exaggerated moves to expel innocuous substances.

Although little studied in the United States, quite a number of experimental examinations done in Europe and Japan point to pollen's immune-strengthening qualities. Dr. Peter Hermus of the University of Vienna, for example, conducted a study of twenty-five women with inoperable uterine cancer. Some were given bee pollen and chemotherapy, others only chemotherapy. Those who received the bee pollen bonus "exhibited a higher concentration of cancer-fighting immune system cells, their antibody production increased, and the level of their infection-fighting and oxygen-carrying red blood cells markedly improved."[62] Other studies show bee pollen revitalizing flagging immune systems by helping people bounce back from surgery. This is why Dr. Naum Ioyrsh, chief of the former Soviet Academy of Vladivostok, calls bee pollen, "one of the original treasure houses of nutrition and medicine."[63]

HONEY

Honey also has a positive effect on immunity. Health researcher Brenda Adderly remarks, "Honey...has been clearly established as a highly effective topical antibiotic, especially useful as a dressing for post-surgical wounds, burns, and other infections."[64] Aside from acting beneficially as a healer, when taken internally honey kills off *H. pyloria* bacteria, which is responsible for stomach ulcers.

PROPOLIS

Propolis was mentioned as another component of raw honey. It is used as a hive sealant by bees who make it by blending sap from trees with their own secretions. Propolis has long been used to support immunity in its fight against unwanted organisms from bacteria to fungi to viruses. Two recent studies, one published in *Drugs Under Experimental and Clinical Research* and one in *Cancer Detection and Prevention*, show it to possess "anti-inflammatory" properties and to be able to "enhance immune response."[65] A single-blind study reported in *Phytomedicine* (2000) compared ninety men and women with genital herpes, treating separate groups with a placebo, propolis, or the commercially marketed herpes drug Zovirax. Propolis proved the most effective treatment of the three.[66]

ROYAL JELLY

This is a milky substance produced by bees after eating pollen. It is fed to the Queen. The proteins, minerals, and vitamins that go into it make it a strong opponent of fungi, viruses, and bacteria. Dr. A. Saenz of the Institut Pasteur in a paper on the therapeutic effects of this substance, looked to its value in treating ulcers, saying that panothenic acid, which is one of the compounds found in the jelly, is useful in that it is necessary "in the protection of the mucosa and the healing of ulcerations."[67] Dr. H. Schmidt, lecturing the German Medical Association on royal jelly, sees it as aiding in blood circulation and cell repair.

Thus, including these bee products in your diet is one means of giving your immunity a good push in the right direction.

DHEA (DIHYDROEPIANDROSTERONE)

DHEA is a key chemical in the functioning of the adrenal gland. It is a precursor to the hormones cortisone and adrenaline. If these are used beyond normal functioning, as in periods of high stress, DHEA will be depleted in the body. And this leads onto weakened immunity, seeing as lack of DHEA brings on a reduction of salivary IgA, an antibody that fights infection in the gastrointestinal tract.

Numerous articles have detailed the chemical's immune-activating ability. An animal study published in the *Journal of Endocrinology* showed supplementation with DHEA protected mice from lethal infections with a whole string of viruses, bacteria, and parasites.[68] Meanwhile an in-vitro study in the *Journal of Immunology* noted DHEA increased the cytotoxicity (that is, killing power) of various antibodies that battle germs.[69] These studies as well as research done on humans indicate the value of this so-called "Mother of All Hormones."

If blood levels are low, 5 mg a day can safely be taken as a supplement.

LACTOFERRIN

Lactoferrin is an iron-binding protein. That means that if excess iron is found in the system, the lactoferrin will take it up and keep it from doing harm. Excess iron is bad because it creates "harmful reactions such as generating free radicals and the pervasive stimulation on infectious agents—such as harmful bacteria, yeast, and viruses—whose metabolic processes rely heavily on iron."[70] Lactoferrin is our main binder of iron, holding it until it is needed for other actions. Thus, lactoferrin is a valuable adjunct to the immune system in that it holds in check the development of pathogens.

It can be obtained in pill form by taking whey protein supplements, since these contain about 0.5 percent lactoferrin. When one is sick, taking about 300 mg a day of lactoferrin is recommended.

MAGNESIUM

Like lactoferrin, which is vital to the body's use of iron, magnesium is key in the body's use of calcium, and this impacts on the immune, circulatory, and nervous system. Medical research has shown magnesium use to be associated with a reduced risk of high blood pressure, osteoporosis, and coronary heart disease.[71]

Leafy green vegetables are one of the best sources for magnesium. Nuts, seeds, avocados, and turnips also contain significant amounts. Other sources include whole grains, legumes, organic eggs, raw milk, carob, honey, and blackstrap molasses.

The recommended daily intake of magnesium is 350 mg, but 800–1,200 mg may be a more realistic figure for obtaining optimum health. Sufficient amounts of magnesium can be obtained from a diet utilizing some of the foods listed above.

VITAMIN A

Vitamin A is essential to immune responsiveness, and has shown particular strength in increasing liver activity. Studies focused on the positive aspects of A supplementation have shown that "vitamin A may boost immune response in the elderly...patients who have undergone surgery, and persons with parasitic infection."[72] Studies on the negative side, that is, ones that show a link between vitamin A deficiency and disease have linked breast cancer, colon cancer, and lung cancer to low levels of vitamin A in the body.

While the vitamin is abundant in carrots, it is present in even higher concentrations in such green leafy vegetables as beet greens, spinach, and broccoli. Yellow or orange vegetables are also good sources. The National Research Council recommends 5,000 IU of vitamin A daily, which amount is easily obtainable through food. As an additional supplement A may be increased during periods of disease, but this should only be done under the direction of a physician since high doses of vitamin A can be harmful.

VITAMIN B6 (pyridoxine)

Vitamin B6 is known to assist in the production of red blood cells and enhance immune response. A significant article in *Biochemical and Biophysical Research Communications* noted that experimental subjects administered B6 showed an increase in levels of T4 lymphocytes. The increase was especially noticeable when B6 was given in conjunction with the Coenzyme Q10, In the body this coenzyme provides a base on which enzyme reactions take place, and B6 is vital for its creation. So, it makes sense that the two of them together would accentuate immune function.[73]

B6 can be found in Brewer's yeast, brown rice, bananas, and pears, which should be a part of your diet. Most of one's required B6 can be consumed in this food, but I would recommend supplementing this with a 50 mg capsule daily.

VITAMIN C (Ascorbate)

In my (Null's) article, "The Antioxidant Vitamin: Vitamin C," I detail some of the immune-empowering effects of this overachieving vitamin. As I note, "Vitamin C assists the immune system in two of its primary functions to rid the body of foreign invaders and to monitor the system for any sign of tumor cells."[74] It does this primarily by stimulating the production of white blood cells. As a component of collagen, a glue that binds cells together into tis-

sues, C forms a first line of defense for collagen is part of the skin and ep-
ithelial lining of the body's orifices where pathogens gain entry. It also stimulates the detoxifying enzymes in the liver, supercharging that organ to carry
out its cleansing work.

A host of studies testify to vitamin C's capacities. For instance, one appearing in the book *Vitamin Intake and Health* looked at the immediate effects
of C. Healthy adults were given one gram intravenously. One hour later lymphocyte production was upped "significantly....[Vitamin C] has been shown
to decrease bacteriological activity."[75] A study of 260 adults with hepatitis
A were given 300 mg of C for several weeks. Their immune systems revived.
Researchers remarked that vitamin C "exerts a remarkable immuno-modulating action."[76]

The Food and Nutrition Board recommends a daily C dose of 45 mg, and
this can easily be obtained from foods, such as oranges and other citrus
fruits, sprouts, berries, tomatoes, sweet potatoes, and green leafy vegetables.
In cases of infection, large dosages can be utilized, under the guidance of a
healthcare practitioner. The major side effects complained of by those who
take mega-doses are "gastrointestinal stress, including cramps, diarrhea, and
nausea. These symptoms, which are caused by acidity rather than ascorbate
itself, seem to disappear when the buffered form of C is taken."[77]

VITAMIN E

Vitamin E helps maintain the health and integrity of cells. It also provides
protection against oxidation. As noted, oxidation occurs when free radical
molecules shoot around the body, bouncing off and damaging other
molecules. As is well known, vitamin C traps these radicals and hence guards
the body from damage. Vitamin E has a similar protective function; however,
as has been recently shown, where C is helpful to many cells, E seems particularly concerned with defending immune system cells. A 1998 study by
Dr. Byung Yu, et al. found "dietary vitamin E to protect against oxidative
damage to DNA in human lymphocytes and white blood cells."[78]

Nutritionists and doctors recommend an adult daily dosage of between
300 to 400 IU. Dietary sources of the vitamin include wheat germ and wheat
germ oil, as well as whole grains, nuts, and seeds.

ZINC

The mineral zinc is important for keeping the body in a state of balance,
maintaining the blood at the proper acidity, removing toxic metals, and aid-

ing the kidneys in seeing there is a healthy equilibrium of metals in the blood flow.

Numerous scientific studies have linked zinc intake to optimum immune function. Let's cite a few.

Since immune responsiveness declines with age, a number of significant investigations have evaluated zinc supplementation on older populations. An experiment by Cristina Fortes, et al., published in 1998 looked at 178 people in an elderly care home in Rome. They were divided into those getting a placebo, and those getting zinc and vitamin A together, or the vitamin or mineral alone. Although results showed that the treated received little of benefit from the vitamin, immune function improved noticeably for those who took zinc supplementation. For them, there was "an increase in total lymphocyte production, and a higher IG antibody response," among other heightenings.[79] A more theoretical study, also concerned with an aged population, noted why zinc has this ability to potentiate immunity. Mocchegian et al. explain that "zinc influences immune cells directly by increasing the activity of multiple enzymes required for DNA replication."[80] This is to say, the production of certain immune cells is dependent on the presence of zinc and without it fewer lymphocytes will be created. As we age, the pool of zinc in the body decreases, and this partially accounts for the body's weakened immunity. Further studies have linked the beneficent action of zinc to the part it plays in fine-tuning leukocytes responsiveness to invasive pathogens, its encouragement of quick response to the first appearance of parasites, its involvement in T cell maturation and differentiation, and its antioxidant qualities.[81] Zinc has proven itself one of the greatest mineral champions of the immune system.

The daily zinc requirement for adults is 20 to 25 mg. It can be taken in capsule form, and also derived from sesame, sunflower, and pumpkin seeds.

Gary Null's Immune Booster and Anti-biowarfare Regimens

You've now gone through a rather daunting, if encouraging list of various herbs and nutritional supplements that provide immune enhancement. At the end of Part III, simply in order to give more salience to these recommendations, we will imagine a case of bioterrroist attack, and see what part alternative therapies and supplements would take in a crisis situation. However, I think it would also be helpful if I presented my own regimens, one for a generalized spurring of the immune system, and another that is primarily antiviral and antibacterial that would be recommended for anyone who might have been exposed to a deadly pathogen.

GARY'S IMMUNE BOOSTER REGIMEN

DAILY RECOMMENDATIONS (mg = milligrams)

colloidal silver	200 parts/million, 20 drops
coenzyme Q10	100 mg, 3 times a day
green tea	3 mg
rosemary	200 mg
alpha-lipoic acid	200 mg, 4 times a day
glutathione	500 mg, divided dose
N-Acetyl-L-Cysteine (NAC)	1,000 mg, divided dose

Trimethylglycine (TMG)	200 mg
Selenium	200 micrograms
Zinc	30 mg
Vitamin C	5,000 mg, divided dose
bioflavonoid	2,000 mg
lycopene	30 mg
grape seed extract	200 mg

GARY'S ANTIMICROBIAL REGIMEN

DAILY RECOMMENDATIONS

aloe vera	3 oz, 3 times a day
astragalus	200 mg
echinacea	200 mg
enteric-coated oil of peppermint	as directed
olive leaf	as directed
oil of oregano	as directed
oil of cinnamon	as directed

Alternative Therapies with an Emphasis on Immune Boosting and Anxiety Alleviation

In other places, we have discussed many alternative therapies that have proven valuable in immune boosting and de-stressing. Here, in keeping with our crucial subthemes, we will note especially those that have a decidedly democratic bent as well as those that involve group activity.

ACUPRESSURE

In ancient China, "when stones and arrows were the only implements of war, many soldiers wounded on the battlefield reported that symptoms of disease that had plagued them for years had suddenly vanished."[82] Physicians were perplexed by the phenomenon. Eventually, they came to see that pressure exerted against parts of the body could be used to temper or conquer certain illnesses and anxiety states. From their observations, they developed a Chinese medical practice called acupressure.

Let's say something first about traditional Chinese beliefs and then about how this practice fits in with more modern beliefs.

The Chinese see the body has an energy field. This energy, called *chi*, runs down meridians, which cross at local points. Some of these are also trigger points, from which energy is conveyed to other parts of the body. Pressure on a local point will bring relief to stresses centered at that bodily area. Pressure on a trigger point will be beneficial to another part of the body (not the one pressed) as this other part is fed energy through the channel passing there. All traditional Chinese therapies (and martial arts, for that matter) are imbued with this philosophy. Tai chi, acupuncture, qi gong, and other practices are concerned with stimulating these points whether by direct touch or choreographed exercise.

If we look at this from a Western perspective, we can follow the thought of Dr. Michael Reed Gach, who writes that if a certain area of the body is damaged or infected, a gentle pressure "triggers the release of endorphins, which are the neurochemicals that relieve pain. As a result, pain is blocked and the flow of blood and oxygen to the affected areas increases."[83] Those familiar with acupuncture will see the parallelism here. Acupuncture, by using a needle to break into the skin, also causes increased blood flow to the affected area. In both cases, a rerouting of blood circulation is believed to draw more immune system cells, which flow in the blood, to the site to boost healing.

Beyond the repair of injured tissue, acupressure is set to deal with the relief of muscle tension and anxiety. As a matter of fact, the two go together. A person under stress will tense his or her muscles in preparation for fight or flight, the instinctive animal reactions to danger. However, since the civilized human usually doesn't carry through on these actions—the worker who is told to hurry up by his supervisor usually doesn't run out of the office or punch the bully in the nose—these tensings remain as cramps in the muscles. They usually correspond to an inability to unwind and release the correspondent mental strain. Recurrent muscle tension builds up toxins around the muscles and interferes with immune function. Acupressure acts to breaks up these centers of tension, get the muscles to release and find a relaxed state.

One thing about acupressure that makes it like the treatment of Dr. Rush, which we described in our historical section, is that it can be easily taught. One does not have to go to a practitioner weekly, but can easily learn it for use at home. As Dr. Gach says about his own methods, "I have also shown hundreds of my acupressure students, patients, and friends how to use acupressure to relieve ulcer pains, menstrual cramps [and other conditions]."[84] When a patient comes to him, he does not only carry out an acupressure manipulation, but instructs that person on how to continue the treatment on him- or herself. This gives the patient more control over when and where to experience the healing.

As Gach concludes, "Acupressure…continues to be the most effective method for self-treatment of tension-related ailments by using the power and sensitivity of the human hand."[85]

DRUMMING

Compare two people. One spends two hours watching a good movie. One spends two hours trying to write a screenplay. Which of the two will have probably learned more about what it takes to make a satisfying film and what obstacles face those who try to make such a work?

The answer is obvious, but I pose this question to point to this same discrepancy in music. Americans are big consumers of music, spending money and time going to concerts, buying CDs, and watching music videos. This certainly has a place, but the moment a person sits down with an instrument her- or himself the real vitality of music shines through in a way that it never can for the listener. This is why I want to put a short section on drumming among other, more conventional ways to reduce stress.

John Yost, a percussionist who has studied drumming worldwide, working both with djembe drum masters in Africa and Taiko percussionists in Japan, facilitates the development and running of drum circles. These are sessions in which drums are passed out and participants drum together, creating an interweaving group harmony.

It's obvious that human life has a beat, since the rhythm of the heart punctuates all the body's processes. But new research, cited by Yost, indicates that the mind, too, works according to the pulsation of brain waves. If these pulsations are disrupted, stress results. Dr. Barry Quinn's research indicates that "drumming for brief periods can actually change a person's brain wave patterns, dramatically reducing stress."[86]

Certainly, the nexus between music and rhythmical biological processes is yet to be explored in any depth, but just as certainly the body does work in concert with rhythmic pulsations, which Yost and others are exploring.

Another percussion-oriented practitioner is Barry Bittman, MD, who integrates use of the drum circle into a fuller program of alternative and traditional therapies. His feeling is that "coordinated whole person medical interventions result in physical, emotional, and social benefits."[87] For him, it is key that one plays music in a group, since this breaks down barriers between people and builds trust between those who are acting in a joint creative project. Like meditation, drumming takes one out of oneself, and, as Bittmann puts it, "orchestrates our immunity."[88]

HOMEOPATHY

Of all the alternative therapies available, the one that might seem most appropriate to a time of epidemics is that of homeopathy. The reason for this is that the homeopathic doctrine was first formulated during a plague, and it was later put to the test in the many epidemics that took place in the nineteenth and early twentieth centuries. In truth, some say that homeopathy is a practice truly geared to such widespread disease outbreaks, and is less appropriate for handling health problems confined to individuals.

Like Dr. Devèze, who ran the Bush Hill facility in Philadelphia during the 1793 plague, Dr. Samuel Hahnemann, initiator of homeopathy, kept experimenting with different methods when faced with a large disease outbreak. In the late eighteenth century, a wave of scarlet fever swept the German town where he lived. In one family, three out of four children were taken sick. The fourth, who was usually the first to become ill, remained free of the disease. Hahnemann reasoned that since the child had been taking *Belladonna* for an infection of the finger joints, she was in some way protected from the infection.[89]

At first, it might seem that Hahnemann had discovered an untried, natural antibiotic. However, the doctor interpreted the situation differently. To his mind, *Belladonna* was something like an anomalous vaccine. It seemed to create an immune response, priming the body for dealing with scarlet fever infection, but it could be designated "anomalous" in that it was not, like other vaccines would eventually be, prepared from the disease-causing bacteria itself. In modern terms, he would be saying that *Belladonna* and the streptococcus bacteria behind the epidemic shared outer membrane markers that would make the same human antibodies responsive to both. (Note, this is only one type of remedy. Homeopathy also employs formulas that exactly parallel vaccines in that they are made from diseased tissue.)

However, there is a second important finding on Hahnemann's part that will lead us directly to a consideration of whether homeopathy is more valuable during epidemics than at other times. As Hahnemann watched the ravages of disease on various different children, he observed another peculiarity.

> All those affected by the epidemic prevailing at a given time have certainly contracted it from one and the same source and hence are suffering from the same disease; but the whole extent of such an epidemic disease…cannot be learned from one single patient, but is only to be perfectly deduced and ascertained from the sufferings of several patients of different constitutions.[90]

His research showed him that there was a range of reaction among the infected, going from being totally prostrated to barely bothered. This is completely in line with what we said earlier about epidemics hitting individuals with different force depending on the state of their immunity (among other factors). According to Hahnemann's follower Paul Herscu, when meeting a disease outbreak, "the homeopath must carefully take the new and unique symptoms that arise in a group of affected individuals to define the most effective treatment."[91] He or she cannot devise a salutary dose until seeing how the illness manifests in a number of cases. As commentator Todd Hoover, MD, puts it, "Just imagine that this group with the similar disease is actually a single patient. As more patients are treated, more symptoms should become apparent which only serve to further clarify the correct remedy choice."[92]

We can see how this view might disturb more individualized homeopathic prescribing. Say that in a town a single child, just returned from foreign travel, came down with scarlet fever. She is taken to a homeopath for treatment. Because the homeopath would only have one example of the illness to study, he or she would not be able to choose the proper remedy with much perspicuity since such choice is dependent on seeing a wide variety of disease presenters.

For this reason, Hoover argues—although this is not a majority opinion in homeopathy—that individualized homeopathic therapy is wrong-headed. "Generalized homeoprophylaxis, however, represents a significant departure from traditional homeopathic doctrine," which he argues was engineered exclusively for combating epidemics.[93]

Hoover then draws on another point, which was established as a doctrine by later practitioners in a significant revision of the original theory. Where Hahnemann believed that once you had found the proper remedy, such as *Belladonna,* you could confidently battle the epidemic, later prescribers learned that there would have to be some variation in treatment in the course of the outbreak since "epidemics tend to evolve over time and geographic spread."[94]

This makes the situation even more complicated. When facing an outbreak, the homeopath must not only examine enough patients to get an idea of how the pathogen varies according to individual constitution, but also be ready to change remedies as the germ mutates. In Hoover's view, then, in situations where there is no epidemic and such trials can not be run, homeopathy is not useful. "Treating mixed populations for dissimilar diseases with the same prophylactic remedy is simply not homeopathy," in his opinion.[95]

Two more positive considerations can be noted. The first is that, whether homeopathy is valuable in non-epidemic situations or not, it is certainly becomes pertinent when there is spread of a pathogen throughout a population. Though, for the reasons noted, "the homeopathic remedies that may be useful in an epidemic will only become known as we see cases, as the disease progresses."[96]

The second is that Hoover's position is not the majority one. Most practitioners hold that, for example, the child with scarlet fever could be well taken care of with homeopathic remedies. This long discussion on a controversy in the alternative practice has been given more to illustrate the close connection between the development of homeopathy and epidemic illnesses, rather than to disparage the use of individual treatments, which have repeatedly proven efficacious in alleviating ills.

So far, however, we haven't described the essence of homeopathic propyhlaxis. "The underlying principle of homeopathy…is that you can use the same thing to restore balance that created the imbalance."[97] Like a vaccine, "the homeopathic remedy restores health by providing a stimulus to the natural healing mechanisms within us all."[98] Homeopathic author Susan Curtis explains more fully:

> The idea is that you take a particular remedy into your system so that it is ready to act should you come into contact with the corresponding disease. The disease will therefore not get a chance to establish itself.[99]

What seems to be a flaw in this argument is that it implies one has to take homeopathic remedies for every known disease (or at least every one you are likely to encounter) to stay protected. However, in practice, this type of treatment would be used during a disease outbreak, such as occurs during flu season. At other times, homeopathic doses are administered to those showing pre-disease states or anxiety. For instance, those who have been made acutely nervous by recent events would be recommended the homeopathic remedies of pulsatilla or causticum.

We can see, therefore, that homeopathy may have a considerable job to do during a disease outbreak. In our next major division, when we see how alternative therapies would be effectual against anthrax, we will learn more about how homeopathy could be employed.

TAI CHI

Tai chi is a Chinese discipline made up of a patterned sequence of flowing movements that stimulate blood circulation and the *chi* (energy) flux in contrast to a Western exercise regimen, such as aerobic exercise, tai chi is both strictly choreographed and slow.

After a warm-up of stretch exercises, each type of tai chi, such as Chan style or Yang style, goes through a particular set of gentle movements that form a dialogue with nature. (Tai chi is best performed outdoors.) Although there is no increase in intensity in the set, there is a building as different moves spark different *chi* bases.

Moreover, unlike vigorous exercise, the emphasis in tai chi is modulated grace. As my co-author's (Feast's) wife, Nhi Chung, a long time tai chi practitioner, puts it, "In tai chi, the slower, the better. But, also, as people don't realize, the slower, the harder."

Because it is slow, it is a practice that can be done by people of all ages. When Chung, as a young woman, would do the exercise in a public park in Saigon, she observed that a frequent participant was one hundred years old! Even people that are sick can profit from the discipline since it is so relaxed.

Yet, it can be taxing. It is harder when slower because of the stance. Every motion is done in a half crouch, not standing, yet not fully bending, as if one were preparing to leap. The stance is called "chut ma" in Cantonese. Here is the Chinese ideogram:

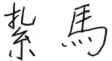

Note that the second ideogram has four strokes at the bottom standing for legs. This is "*ma*," which means horse. The stance, when the arms are raised above the head, is said to resemble a rearing horse.

When Chung first started her practice at age eighteen, going with a childhood friend, the teacher told them to assume the chut ma stance and circle their arms in front of them as if holding a large ball. For one month, all they did was stand, increasing their ability to assume the stance from about five minutes up to a half hour.

As is traditional, the discipline was practiced in a class of about thirty. It is believed that *chi* circulation is heightened and the link to natural surroundings strengthened by working in a group. In this way, individual flow joins to the collective energy tide, which helps the participants center in the universe in a new way.

Alternative Therapies in an Anthrax Attack

We've spent some time specifying the varied herbs, nutrients, and alternative practices that can be used in a proactive attempt to be ready for the appearance of new pathogens. We have spoken of how to strengthen immunity and reduce tension and depression. But this discussion has been necessarily vague in some respects and may well have left you a bit dissatisfied. You may still want more details. If I can hazard a guess at the type of question still in your mind, it might be something like this: "Yes, Gary, I see the importance of what you have said, but I am still worried. What should I do in case terrorists bombard our area with deadly germs?"

So, let's move beyond broad-gauged prescriptions, and imagine a concrete scenario. Let's say you were in an area exposed to anthrax. Would there be any place for alternative medicine in this situation?

As we've seen, Dr. Strauss from the National Center for Complementary and Alternative Medicine (NCCAM) said in no uncertain terms, that alternative therapies have nothing to offer in such circumstances. Powerful diseases, such as anthrax, leave you no time to fiddle around with acupuncture and medicinal herbs, since they strike hard and fast and must be routed immediately There is no time for the slower, milder actions of alternative remedies.

However, as we've shown, and not only in the case of anthrax but in many of the diseases the CDC thinks terrorists might employ, antibiotics are hardly foolproof. Many times they are defeated by the pathogen. In that case, wouldn't it make sense, if a person contracted one of these diseases, to *supplement* the antibiotics or antivirals with a known immune stimulator, as long as the supplement was known not to react with the traditional drug in any perverse way? Moreover, what about the cases, and there are many, where the disease does not respond to any drug and the best the patient can get is supportive care. Wouldn't it be sensible to make part of this care the administration of herbs, vitamins, and other supplements that will empower the immune system to react?

This is what we are going to suggest, then. And remember, use of alternative practices as supplements should never be done sub rosa. The primary physician, who in the anthrax scenario, would be administering traditional drugs, should be consulted about any alternative therapy you are considering. What would seem valuable is to combine traditional and alternative therapies as the most holistic way to confront the emergency.

So how does one handle the anthrax attack mindfully?

First things first. You may remember that at the head of this third part, we remarked that the two factors that determine one's physical reaction to a pathogen is amount of exposure and robustness of constitution. Therefore, one of the keys to weathering such an assault is to minimize contamination. This, as we stated, involves wearing protective garments and keeping everything scrupulously clean. An advisory from the National Center for Homeopathy has this to add for anyone in a exposed position:

> Don't put stuff in your mouth, especially your hands or anything that you or anyone else touches with hands, unless they're washed first. This means don't chew your fingernails or the end of your pencil. Don't eat with your hands unless you have washed them or the food can be held in its wrapper.[100]

If, however, one has been infected with anthrax, supplements can play a part along with antibiotics. Here are my recommendations.

VITAMIN C

Studies have shown that vitamin C is effective against cholera, whooping cough, and tetanus.[101] "Of great interest…is that all three of these infections are associated with very significant microbe-generated toxins, like anthrax."[102]

Thomas Levy, MD, argues that mega doses of the vitamin are called for in case of anthrax infection. "Start vitamin C infusions at up to 700 mg/kg at a time as often as necessary to obtain a positive clinical response." He scoffs at those who say traditional antibiotics will be enough to do the job against this pathogen. "It is absolutely unthinkable not to try it [vitamin C] or add it to whatever protocol is being administered to the patient."[103] He notes further that anthrax rapidly metabolizes the C, and so the body is in constant need of more C when striving against the infection.

ECHINACEA

Echinacea will foster the production of more white blood cells (that is, antibodies) when these are lowered due to their engagement in combating an infection. "During the period of infection, when the body is running low on its resources, echinacea has been found to have a strong and direct activating force on the body's ability to produce macrophages and speed them to the area of infection."[104]

For this anthrax infection, echinacea should be taken as a liquid extract, one half to one teaspoon three times a day for seven to ten days.

GARLIC

Garlic, as noted, is an all-around immune helper, boosting the production of antibodies and attacking a wide range of pathogens. In truth, its germ-fighting abilities seem to put it in a class by itself. In scientific studies, "garlic was found to be a more potent antibiotic than penicillin, ampicillin, doxycycline, streptomycin, and cephalexin."[105]

As a supplement when fighting off the pathogen, one can take the same dose noted previously. Eat one clove (after crushing it) three times a day.

VITAMIN A

Just as an infected person uses up his or her store of vitamin C quickly, so the patient's vitamin A levels plummet. Therefore, "the body's need for vitamin A increases dramatically when it is under attack."[106] For this reason alone, aside from vitamin A's ability to fortify immunity, it should be taken by the sufferer.

One should go above the usual recommendation 5,000 IU daily, although, since vitamin A can have harmful side effects. Exact dosage should be determined in consultation with your health practitioner.

BETA CAROTENE

Beta carotene is another immune system assistant, and not only does it enhance immunity by activating T cells and B cells, but it works in tandem with vitamin A.

A normal dose of beta carotene would be 60 milligrams daily, but this should be upped, in consultation with your healthcare provider when battling this infection.[107]

HYDRATION

Levy also remarks on the need for hydration, that is, large intake of water, from two to four quarts daily. This will not only augment vitamin C therapy, but will compensate for the high water loss that takes place in anthrax sufferers.[108]

HOMOEPATHIC MEASURES

Although one can take various homeopathic remedies to deal with the different symptoms of anthrax, the most important preparation is anthracinum. Like vaccines, this is made by taking elements of the disease itself and treating in a way that makes them of benefit to the body.[109]

For an adult, the dose would be one dose of 30x potency, once a day for three days. A child can take one dose once.

A number of other herbs with immune-strengthening properties have been suggested for use in this context, and they can be taken, although they are not as absolutely vital as the ones noticed in our list. These would be Chinese ginseng, astragalus, licorice root, pau d'arco, wild indigo, myrrh, thyme, and oil of oregano.

Conclusion

SELF AND COMMUNITY ONE AND THE SAME?

We've said that one of the founders of sociology, Emile Durkheim, maintained that the human being had crossed tendencies: one urge to act for personal benefit, one to act for the collective good.

We want to move now to the thought of another early figure of social science, because he looked at the same doubleness from a different angle.

In G. H. Mead we find a more attractive thesis: that the personal side of humans, the self, is the product of collective life and remains tied to it in every moment. For Mead, there is no such divorce as Durkheim imagined between the strands in a human personality, because the collective side is at all times dominant. He puts this pithily, "It is important to recognize the self, as one among other individuals, is not subjective, nor are its experiences as such subjective."[1]

We take up Mead's thought here, not as a corrective to Durkheim, but to help us in our final consideration of the individual's relation to the collective in a time of upheaval and phase transition. Since this is a book that offers advice, and we have already spoken on physical and mental changes that can be made to bolster health, it is now time to speak about spirit-enhancing action in the community. But to give such advice, we need some grasp of what a human being actually is.

We proceed in three steps. We begin by giving attention to a fuller exposition of Mead's thoughts, which may seem paradoxical at this point. Then we turn to Pascal to see how he, taking a similar view of the self to Mead, analyzed the problems facing a person in a time of paradigm shift. We see that it was his own movement away from a collective, that led Pascal to despair. On the other hand, turning for a last time to the yellow fever outbreak in Philadelphia, we learn that those who embraced a collective ethos, not only escaped despair, but resolved the quandary of paradigm clash. We end with a few recommendations.

In his lectures at the University of Chicago at the turn of the nineteenth century, Mead often brought up the example of two men fencing. A fencer "may deliberately feint to open up a place of attack," he said.[2] Let's think about what is entailed in a feint. The beginning of an offensive stroke is started to throw the opponent off guard. To do this, the attacker must be able to accurately imagine how the defender will act. Ideally, this means he must not only be able to judge how that defender will act physically, but know how he judges the attacker. Unless he knows what the defender thinks of him, he cannot guess if he will expect a feint at this moment or not.

Ultimately, Mead asserts the origin of self is from situations such as these.

He makes his argument in this way. Nothing can be known unless it is first distinguished from what is around it. The first stage of understanding is to get straight that the thing to be analyzed is separate from everything else. Then, to know ourselves, to know that we possess individuality, we have to be able to separate ourselves from others. Mead's primal contention is this. We can only obtain this separation of the self by imagining how we are seen from other's eyes. "It is the social process of influencing others in a social act and then taking the attitude of the others aroused by the stimulus [such as the feint], and then reacting in turn to this response, which constitutes a self."[3]

This is hardly the place for a full discussion of Mead's thought. Suffice it to say that, by studying such things as how children play games, he is able to make a good case for the idea that we acquire our sense of self by seeing how we look to others.

The upshot is that any attempt by a person to separate from his or her surrounding community to exist in total self reliance will end up, not enhancing but attenuate individuality, since it will be severing it from its basis.

We can follow this out by seeing how Pascal, when broken off from the religious group that had given him sustenance, declined into a deeply pessimistic attitude.

PASCAL AND COMMUNITY

Let us begin with a startling anticipation of Mead's views in Pascal.

> Not content with our own proper and individual life, we want to live an imaginary life in the mind of others [*"dans l'idées des autres d'une vie imaginaire"*], and to this end we struggle to make a show. We labour ceaselessly to improve and preserve our imaginary being, and neglect the real. And if we possess calm, or generosity, or fidelity, we are eager to proclaim them so as to pin these real virtues to our fictitious being, and we would gladly strip them from the real to add them to the other.[4]

The tone is totally opposed to Mead's, while the thought is similar. For Mead, it is inevitable and generative that we live in the minds of others; while for Pascal the same fact reflected humans vanity. To see why Pascal's view was so at odds with Mead's, we have to examine his changing connection to the community.

At first, we might think the marked change in Pascal's writing came from his immersion in (fruitless) attempts to convert unbelievers. We've seen that in Mead a person learns by (mentally) taking another's position. This type of behavior, the sociologist argues, eventually gives birth to thought, which is an internal conversation between an imagined other and the self. Pascal's *Pensées,* written to convince doubters of the truths of Catholicism, displays something like Mead's idea of the mental colloquy. In the book Pascal constantly puts words in the mouth of an imagined free thinker whom he is striving to persuade to his viewpoint.

Although the unbeliever never gets the upper hand, one feels that by taking his part, Pascal is weakening his own faith, since his view of human nature here is many degrees darker than it is in the earlier *Provincial Letters.* We will see in a minute, though, that such a supposition is misguided.

In the earlier text, Pascal depicted the Jesuits as dangling temptation in front of their confessants by allowing them to excuse venial (or even mortal) sins. In the *Pensées,* though, there is no need for Jesuits. By this I mean, in the later work, humans exhibit a rooted tendency to rationalize errors so as to avoid responsibility for them, and just as generally ignore their duties in favor of chasing a round of pleasures.

> The one thing that consoles us for our miseries is diversion, and yet that is the greatest of our miseries [*"c'est la plus*

> *grande de nos misères"]*. For it is this that mainly checks
> consideration of ourselves and ruins us unconsciously.
> Without it we should fall into ennui, and ennui should
> drive us to seek a better way out.[5]

An apt and powerful parable helps Pascal point up what he sees as the absurdity of humans' persistent misdirection of attention.

> Whence comes it that this man who lost his only son a few
> months ago, and who this very morning was overwhelmed
> with lawsuits and quarrels, has now forgotten all about
> them? Be not surprised: he is absorbed in watching where
> the boar will pass which his hounds have been hunting so
> hotly all day.[6]

We've said it might seem that the more dyspeptic view of humankind found in this final work of Pascal's stems from his attempt to understand the mind of an unbeliever. However, a moment's thought about the addressees and the trying circumstances of each work will give us a clue to a more plausible interpretation.

As noted, the *Provincial Letters*, were written to defend the harried Jansenists sect. The theme is how the Jansenists *as a body* were being attacked by the Jesuit group. Remember I spoke of how he read each letter to his fellow Jansenists for approbation? So, no matter how embattled the group was, Pascal was working in sync with them, fighting for them, living in deep solidarity.

Things had changed by the time of the *Pensées*. The Jesuits had obtained an even stronger position with the Pope, who would soon break up the Jansenists nunnery and disperse the religious group forever. However, that was not key. What affected Pascal even more was that the Jansenists were fighting among themselves, many saying they should stop defending their leader and agree with whatever the Jesuits said, to preserve their lives.

Pascal felt this was insupportable, but more and more fell away from the strong position he espoused. The philosopher called them to his rooms for a last ditch effort to convince them to stay the course. Here is the heart-rending way Pascal biographer Ernest Mortimer describes the situation:

> A meeting was arranged in Pascal's rooms as he was too ill
> to attend elsewhere. The situation was reviewed and Pascal

rose to speak. After a few powerful sentences, he faltered, lost the thread and fell senseless. The room was cleared and he was brought back to consciousness. He explained to Gilberte, "I saw these men, trustees of the truth, caving in; and it finished me."

For this brief...interlude, Pascal was almost alone.[7]

We argue that the profound melancholy that fills this last work of the French genius is the product of a loss of community. As he struggled to fit the church to the new scientific world view, he was saddled with a deeply embittered perspective because he seemed to have been deserted. Facing the intellectual instability at a time of phase transition was almost unbearable without a community of like-minded seekers beside him.

But what if the situation is faced in tandem? Will the negotiation of the difficult period be any less harsh? Perhaps another look at Philadelphia can set us on the right path to answer these questions.

PHILADELPHIA: COMMUNITY AND PARADIGM

We ended the last discussion of Philadelphia with a paradox. It seemed the impromptu government, and, more significantly, the new, streamlined, radical democratic methods of that government, did not endure after the crisis because a rationale for keeping intact these innovations did not exist. The methods used by this default state were ones that tied up with a new world view which had not been worked out yet. But, still, as the paradox stressed, even with no elaborated framework, the major elements of this problematic were gingerly put into practice.

But how is that possible?

We would make this argument. The epidemic, by dissolving all the normal patterns overnight, created a new network between people. At first, those who remain are scared witless, but then things change. The best description we have of this feeling at the time comes in a work by Mathew Carey, who lived in the Philadelphia during the yellow fever outbreak and published an account of the event barely a month after it had ended. He makes this extraordinary comparison.

There has been a strong analogy between the state of Philadelphia, and that of an army. About the close of August... an universal trepidation benumbed people's

> faculties.... Just so, with an army of recruits.... But [once
> they have been] familiarized...with the horrid trade of
> death, the obstinate phalanx beholds unmoved, its ranks
> mowed down and death advancing.... Even thus it was
> here.... When the horrors of the scene were constantly in-
> creasing...then people cast away their various preventa-
> tives.... And then it was, that they assumed a manly
> fortitude, tempered with the sober, serious pensiveness,
> befitting such an awful scene.[8]

Like an army, the citizens were experiencing danger as a unit, and like an army, they gained a special sense of informal unity, unknown in normal circumstances.

It was not only those who staffed the ad-hoc city government or worked at Bush Hill, certainly the leading appreciators of the change, who experienced this communion. As Carey points out, it extended both to individuals and to those at a distance.

Small groups, such as those running the almshouse, and individuals, affected by the unprecedented crisis, acted in ways that showed a deep love for their fellows, which could not appear as such in average times. "Amidst the general abandonment of the sick that prevailed," Carey wrote,

> there were to be found many illustrious instances of men
> and women, some in the middle, others in the lower
> spheres of life, who, in the exercise of the duties of human-
> ity, exposed themselves to dangers, which terrified men,
> who have hundreds of times faced death without fear, in
> the field of battle.[9]

Simultaneously, places at a distance were also rising to the occasion. "The sympathy for our calamities, displayed in various places [that is, other towns], and the very liberal contributions raised for our relief, reflect the highest honor on their inhabitants, and demand our warmest gratitude."[10] While cities like New York, were closing their doors, not just to people fleeing Philadelphia but to goods from that port, others offered refuge and succor to the escapees, ignoring the danger of contagion.

Yes, people change in a crisis. This is nothing new. But the assertion we are making is this. That a different sense of community, involving an intuitive ascertainment of the truth of Mead's thought, that our self is the product of our community, leads people to live *an anticipatory life*. That is to say, they begin operating and recreating the city in a way that corresponds to a new, previously unlived paradigm.

Perhaps, this is not always true, but in the cases we are discussing, the one facing us and the one facing Philadelphia, the emergent world view is one with more liberal strictures. As we've shown, for Philadelphia, the temporary society was more humane, more equalitarian, more free, and resolutely put people over property. When the crisis was over, society lapsed back into a less estimable way of doing things.

Eventually, of course, the new way of seeing did take hold and a new world view was embraced. This is not inevitable. It is possible for a society to stagnate for long periods. All we want to indicate is that if a new framework takes hold, it can come about in two ways, following two time sequences. It can arise glacially, through the piecemeal elaboration of a position in various places, such as universities, laboratories, and restricted political arenas; or it can happen instantly, when a people under the pressure of death forges a default proto state (or the equivalent).

It takes a community effort to move with dispatch to a higher level.

ADVICE ON COMMUNITY INVOLVEMENT

This said, we can restate one of our unifying themes in this way. We are now in a period of phase transition between the older medical model, which sees the body at war with pathogens, and the newer medical model, which sees pathogens, body, and environment forming complex configurations that can turn beneficial or harmful.

When you choose a way of taking care of your health, you are implicitly taking up one of these models. And these models do not only contain intellectual constructs of disease process, but social relations. In these later terms, the choice is between being under the endless tutelage of a doctor or of educating oneself about health, so as to be an equal participant in care for your own well being.

Consciousness is all. When a patient, say, a man with lung problems, goes to a hidebound, traditional doctor, he wants to be unconscious. He doesn't want to think about either the sickness or what he has done to encourage it. By contrast, if this man went to a alternative practitioner, he would go wanting to be as aware as possible. He would desire to understand his disease, what part his life patterns have taken in promoting it, and see how he can alter his own activities to preclude recurrences. This is a first stage.

A real, deep awareness goes beyond knowledge into conviction. My vegetarian friend, whom I found outside McDonalds, intellectually knew he was wrong, but he didn't know it forcefully enough to be convinced of what he knew. A second stage consciousness entails both comprehension and action on the comprehension.

Yet, going above this, there is also a third level, being conscious of how what you believe in connects to the larger movements of history. Of course, you can know and abide by health practices that fall under the new medical paradigm and not see what you are doing in light of the phase transition. However, once you see that each choice is either an endorsement or a repudiation of a world view, it follows that you will act to advance your favored perspective.

If you are aligned with the newer paradigm, you will feel compelled to do such things as forming or joining groups, like the one Walene James created to disseminate information on vaccines, that help make the new perspective (shut out of much discussion) available. You will get information (and encourage others to get information) from alternate media, which try to give a wider spectrum of views. You will go to rallies or teach-ins to support just causes that are another reflection of this shift. All in all, this means tying yourself into a web of those who are trying to change the world, rather than lying back and letting that world wash over you.

Otherwise you are not fully aware and moving concurrently in every linked dimension: physical, mental, and social, to make your world and yourself health-bound.

Coda

[President] Clinton began asking his friends, cabinet members, even House Speaker Newt Gingrich whether they had read the book and what they had thought about it. After a White House meeting on another topic, the president suddenly turned to John Hamre, the deputy secretary of defense, and asked whether he could speak to him privately for a few moments. As the two men walked into the Oval Office, Clinton said he had recently read *The Cobra Event* and asked Hamre whether the novel's scenario was plausible.

We began with two scary incidents that should have created trepidation in the mind of our readers. We end with two ways of finding hope, one in a famous novel by an honor-laden *New Yorker* writer, one by an obscure, underground poet, whose reputation among the cognoscenti has been building for decades, but who is invisible to the larger culture.

Richard Preston's *The Cobra Event* caught President Clinton's eye and rocketed to the top of the best-seller list. It is the story of how the government (FBI, CDC, and other agencies) faces off against a lone terrorist who is spreading a bioengineered virus, made of equal parts: the common cold, smallpox, and butterfly brainpox.

As in other techno-thrillers, that are written within the older paradigm, hope is seen as arising from progress in hard science. It is assumed that if we just invent a new gadget, we can handle anything. So throughout the novel, one reads loving descriptions of such things as a machine "that could throw a beam of infrared laser light on an object and then analyze the spectrum of the light bouncing off the object."[1] Then there are the Felix machines, which can decipher the DNA codes of presented biological materials, the electron microscopes, the X-ray diffraction machines, and, of course, all manners of heavy artillery.[2]

Preston interviewed many heavies in law enforcement, bioterrorist response, and the handling of medical emergencies, and his book is strongly colored by their views. For them, technical wizardry gives the strongest assurance that we can face the bioterrorism threat with confidence.

Steve Dalachinsky in his poem, "the phone call (first)," offers hope of a less lofty kind.[3] Dalachinsky lives perhaps twenty blocks from the World Trade Center. On the morning of September 11, 2001, he was puttering around his house, radio and TV off. He received a call from a friend in Paris, who was watching the news and wanted to know about the attack.

In a book of poems, *Morir Soñando [to die dreaming]: poems of 9/11, etc.*, Dalachinsky mediates on the United States after the WTC trauma. But he does not troll for illusory hopes of technical mastery as a way to assuage his fears. Instead, there is the quirky, resilient attempt to face the new, grim situation, in which there is such a divide from the pre–September 11 days that it is as if everything is happening for the first time. When his wife Yuko tremblingly asks about anthrax and when a wide range of insomnias and tics appear among his friends, he goes forward with a keen edge of observation which doesn't flinch at a naked rendering of his soul. In his stanzas, it is the human ability to gradually make peace with the dead and slowly tread forward with a heavier but wiser heart that signifies our indomitable spirit and gives us reason to suspect we will endure.

The poem is too long to quote in full, but I think it might be appropriate to end with an excerpt.

Steve Dalachinsky

THE PHONE CALL (FIRST)

———

i place a call   expecting to get a machine   i get a real person instead
it's a woman   i hang   up
i step into the hall   i've been expecting a call from a friend   i miss it

this is not the first time this has happened   yet it is…

it's the first star i've seen since the towers collapsed
it used to be hidden behind them
the first moon
blossoming between the chimney
& the water tower…

it's not the same   nothing will ever be the same   so what's the rush

sleep   sleep as much as you want   everyone sleeps a lot now   sleep late
sleep as late as you want   everyone oversleeps   & oversleeps
they're depressed & anxious   they'd rather have good dreams
being late for work has become fashionable—   what's the rush

what's anthrax   she asks me like a little girl—don't bother me i'm playing the game

you'll know it when you catch it
i proclaim   & by that time it won't matter
i'm afraid i say   & i'm not afraid to say it   i'm afraid & everybody knows it

i make phone calls hoping to get machines

i hope the voice on the other end
did not feel frightened   when I suddenly hung up

things are different now
from today on   everything must be abridged.

———

Resource List

(These are in addition to works listed in the notes.)

BIOWARFARE

PRINT

Atlas, R. M., "Combating the Threat of Bioterror and Biowarfare: Defending Against Biological Weapons is Critical to Global Security," *Bioscience*, June 1999.

British Medical Association, *Biotechnology, Weapons, and Humanity* (Amsterdam: Harwood, 1999).

Eitzen, E. M., Jr. "Education Is the Key to Defense Against Bioterrorism," *Ann. Emerg. Med.*, August 1999, 34 (2): 221–3.

Henderson, D. A., "The Looming Threat of Bioterrorism," *Science*, February 26, 1999, 283 (9254): 1279–82.

Kortepeter, M. H., et al., "Bioterroism," *Journal of Environmental Health*, January 2001, 63 (3): 21–24.

Lederber, J., ed., *Biological Weapons: Limiting the Threat* (Cambridge, MA: MIT Press, 1999).

Rotx, L. D., et al., "Bioterrorism Preparedness: Planning for the Future," *J Public Health Manag Pract.*, July 2000, 6 (4): 45–9.

Simon, J. D. "Biological Terrorism, Preparing to Meet the Threat," *JAMA*, August 6, 1997, 278 (5): 428–30.

Voelker, R. "Bioweapons Preparedness Chief Discusses Priorities in World of 21st-Century Biology," *JAMA*, 2992, 283: 573–75.

Zilinskas, R. A., "Iraq's Biological Weapons: The Past As Future?" *JAMA*, 1997, 278: 418–24.

WEB

AMA Disaster Preparedness and Medical Response site
http://www.ama-assn.org/go/disasterpreparedness

CDC public health emergency preparedness and response site
http://www.bt.cdc.gov/

Center for Mental Health Services, "Mental Health Aspects of Terrorism."
http://www.mentalhealth.org/publications/allpubs/KEN-01-0095/
default.asp

Center for the Study of Bioterrorism and Emerging Infections
http://www.slu.edu/colleges/sph/bioterrorism

eMedicine: Information on grief and bereavement, and topics related
to bioterrorism
http://www.emedicine.com

FDA Bioterrorism page
http://www.fda.gov/oc/opacom/hottopics/bioterrorism.html

Holistic-online "Bioterrorism Infocenter"
http://www.holisticonline.com/Remedies/Biot/biot-home.htm

Kid's Health site
http://www.kidshealth.org/breaking_news/tragedies.htm.

Texas Medical Assn. Bioterrorism Resource Center
http://www.texmed.org/has/bioterrorism.asp

Your Personal Pharmacist.com, "Bioterrorism: What You Should Know"
http://www.yourperonalpharmacist.com/sys-tmpl/bioterrorismwhat
youshouldknow

ANTHRAX

PRINT

Blate, Michael, "Anthrax and Co.: Some Alternative Treatments," *Townsend Letter for Doctors and Patients*, January 2002.

Davis, J. and Johnson-Winegar, A., "The Anthrax Terror," *Aerospace Power Journal*, Winter 2000, 14 (4): 15–30.

Naslin, D., et al., "Recognition and Treatment of Anthrax," *JAMA*, 1999, 282: 1624–25.

Pile, J. C., et al., "Anthrax as a Potential Biological Warfare Agent," *Archives of Internal Medicine*, March 9, 1998, 158, 429.

WEB

The New England Journal of Medicine;
"Information about Anthrax and Other Biological Threats"
http://nejm.org/specialnotice

ANTIBIOTIC RESISTANCE

WEB

CDC, "Background on Antibiotic Resistance"
http://www.cdc.gov/antibioticresistance

Microbial Research, Global Health, "Antimicrobial Resistance"
http://www.niaid.nih.gov/dmid/antimicrob

IMMUNITY

PRINT

Neu, H. C., "The Body's Defenses Against Infections," in *The Columbia University College of Physicians and Surgeons Complete Home Medical Guide*, 3rd Edition (New York, 1995), Chapter 18.

WEB

NIH, "Understanding the Immune System"
http://rex.nci.nih.gov/PATIENTS/INFO_TEACHER/bookshelf/NIH_immune/index.html

ALTERNATIVE HEALTH

PRINT

Haddad, C., et al., "Assessment of Immune Status of Vegan Versus Non-Vegan Adults," *Nutrition Research Newsletter*, December 1999, 18 (12), 15.

O'Hara, M., et al., "A Review of 12 Commonly Used Medicinal Herbs," *Arch Fam Med*, November/December 1998, 7: 523–36.

"Rev Up Your Immune System to Prevent Disease," *Healthy Immunity Newsletter*, February 2000, 1–4. (Also available online.)

Sayre, J. K., *Ancient Herbs and Modern Herbs: A Comprehensive Reference Guide to Medicinal Herbs, Human Ailments, and Possible Herbal Remedies* (San Carlos, Calif.: Bottlebrush Press, 2001).

Schechter, S., "Power Up with High Energy Herbs," *Better Nutrition*, June 1998.

WEB

Chaitow, L. "Antibiotic Alternatives"
http://www.garynull.com/Documents/Continuum/Antibiotics
Alternatives.htm

HerbMed
http://www.herbmed.org

IBIDS (International Bibliographic Information on Herbal Supplements
http://ods.od.nih.gov/databases/ibids.html

Plants for a Future
http://www.scs.leeds.ac.uk/pfaf/D_intro.html

Phytochemical and Ethnobotanical Databases
http://www.ars-grin.gov/duke

Starbuck, Jamison, "7 Herbs for Women," *Better Nutrition*, December 1998.
http://www.betternutrition.com

Starbuck, Jamison, "Herbs to the Rescue (to Boost Immunity),
Better Nutrition, November 2000
http://www.betternutrition.com

Notes

PREFACE

1. Laurie Garrett, *Betrayal of Trust: The Collapse of Global Public Health* (New York: Hyperion, 2002), 416.
2. Garrett, 418.
3. Ibid.
4. Ibid., 378.
5. William J. Broad and Judith Miller, "Report Provides New Details of Soviet Smallpox Accident, " *New York TImes*, June 15, 2002, A1. See also Judith Miller, Stephen Engelberg, and William Broad, *Germs: Biological Weapons and America's Secret War* (New York: Simon and Schuster, 2001), 231.
6. Broad and Miller, A15.
7. Ibid., 1.
8. Ibid., A15.
9. Miller, et al., *Germs*, 76.

INTRODUCTION

1. Laurie Garrett, *Betrayal of Trust: The Collapse of Global Public Health* (New York: Hyperion, 2002), 515.
2. Ibid., 180.
3. Ibid., 417.
4. Ibid., 483.
5. Michael T. Osterholm and John Schwartz, *Living Terrors: What America Needs to Know to Survive the Coming Bioterrorist Catastrophe* (New York: Delacorte Press, 2001), 129.
6. Garrett, 414.
7. Quoted in ibid., 377.
8. Ibid., 380.
9. Ibid., 456.
10. Quoted in ibid., 457.
11. Gary Null (with James Feast), *AIDS: A Second Opinion* (New York: Seven Stories Press, 2002), 371.
12. Blaise Pascal, *Pensées*, H. F. Stewart, translator (New York: Pantheon, 1950), 135.
13. Ibid., 27.
14. Ibid., 97.
15. Ibid., 151.
16. Emile Durkheim, *The Division of Labor in Society*, W. D. Halls, translator (New York: The Free Press, 1984), [my itals], 56–57.
17. Garrett, 534.
18. Osterholm, 176.
19. Ibid., 173.
20. Garrett, 533–34.

21. It is interesting to note, in the light of our discussion of the collective and individualist layers of personality, that it his hidden confession, Pascal says he is experiencing, "God of Abraham, God of Issac, God of Jacob, not of the philosophers and the scholars." See, Blaise Pascal, "Pascal's Memorial," in *Great Shorter Works of Pascal*, Emile Cailliet and John C. Blankenagel, translators (Philadelphia: The Westminster Press, 1948), 117. As I read Pascal's phrase, it indicates one can have no notion of god simply through intellectual assent. However, don't jump to the conclusion that what is wanted is emotional apprehension of the Godhead. "Abraham," "Issac," "Jacob," these were Old Testament patriarchs. Their god is that of the Jewish people. Pascal indicates that *divinity can only be known when experienced within a collectivity*. For him to build up a less superficial relation to divinity, he would have to follow his younger sister's Jacqueline's footsteps and join a religious community. Jacqueline became a nun. See also Jean Steinmann, *Pascal*, Martin Turnell, translator (New York: Harcourt, Brace, and World, 1965), 82–3.
22. Steinmann, 53.

PART I: BIOLOGICAL WARFARE AND DRUG-RESISTANT GERMS

1. George W. Christopher, Theodore J. Cieslak, Julie A. Pavlin, and Edward M. Eitzen, "Biological Warfare: A Historical Perspective," *JAMA* August 6, 1997, 278 (5), 2. Or: http://jama.ama-assn.org/v278n5/ffull/jsc7044.html.
2. Ibid., 3.
3. Ibid., 6.
4. Laurie Garrett, *Betrayal of Trust: The Collapse of Global Public Health* (New York: Hyperion, 2002), 369.
5. Seán Murphy, Alastair Hay, and Steve Rose, *No Fire, No Thunder: The Threat of Chemical and Biological Weapons* (New York: Monthly Review Press, 1984), 49.
6. Ibid., 53.
7. Ibid., 53–54.
8. Ibid., 56.
9. Judith Miller, Stephen Engelberg, and William Broad, *Germs: Biological Weapons and America's Secret War* (New York: Simon and Schuster, 2001), 31.
10. Garrett, 19.
11. Ibid., Chapter Two: "Landa-Landa."
12. "History of Bioterrorism," in *Biological Terrorism Response Manual*, 8–9. http://www.bioterry.com/History_of_Biological_Terrorism.asp.
13. For further reading on this history, see, "History of Biological Warfare and Current Threat," in *Bioterrorism Preparedness Program*, Environmental Health, Rhode Island Department of Health, http://www.healthri.org/environment/biot/hist.htm.; "History of Biological Warfare," USAMRID, http://www.gulfwarvets.com/biowar.htm.
14. Michael T. Osterholm and John Schwartz, *Living Terrors: What America Needs to Know to Survive the Coming Bioterrorist Catastrophe* (New York: Delacorte Press, 2001), 7.
15. Ibid., 8.
16. Lisa D. Rotz, Ali S. Khan, Scott R. Lillibridge, Stephen M. Ostroff, and James M. Hughes, "Public Health Assessment of Potential Biological Terrorism Agents," *Emerging Infectious Diseases*, February 2002, 8 (2), 1. http://www.cdc.gov/ncidod/EID/vol8no2/01-0164.htm.

17. Ibid., 2.

18. Ibid., 2.

19. L. Shireley, T. Dwelle, and D. Streitz, "Human Anthrax Associated With an Epizootic Among Livestock—North Dakota, 2000," *MMWR*, (*Morbidity and Mortality Weekly Report*) August 17, 2001, 50 (32), 1. http://www.cdc.gov/mmwr/preview/mmwrhtml/mm5032a1.htm.

20. "Inhalational Anthrax," Holistic-online, 1. http://holisticonline.com/Remedies/biot/biot_anthrax-inhalational.htm.

21. Luciana Borio, Dennis Frank, Venkat Mani, Carlos Chirboga, Michael Pollanen, Mary Ripple, Syed Ali, Constance DiAngelo, Jacqueline Lee, Jonathan Arden, Jack Titus, David Fowler, Tara O'Toole, Henry Masur, John Bartlett, and Thomas Inglesy, "Death Due to Bioterrorism-Related Inhalational Anthrax," *JAMA*, November 28, 2001, 286 (20), 2. http://jama.ama-assn.org/issues/v286n20/ffull/joc11802. html. On the victims of the inhalational anthrax attacks, see also, Larry M. Bush, Barry H. Abrams, Anne Beall, and Caroline C. Johnson, "Index Case of Inhalational Anthrax Due to Bioterrorism in the United States," *The New England Journal of Medicine*, November 29, 2001, 345 (22), 1607–10; Bushra Min, J. P. Dym, Frank Kuepper, et al., "Fatal Inhalational Anthrax with Unknown Source of Exposure in a 61-Year-Old Woman in New York City," *JAMA*, February 20, 2002, 287 (7); and "Update: Adverse Events Associated with Anthrax Prophylaxis Among Postal Employees—New Jersey, New York City, and the District of Columbia Metropolitan Area, 2001, *MMWR*, November 30, 2001, 50 (47), 1051–4.

22. "Investigation of Bioterrorism-Related Anthrax, 2001, *MMWR*, December 5, 2001, 286 (21), 2. http://jama.ama-assn.org/issues/v286n21/ffull/jwrl205-1.html.

23. Rhode Island Department of Health, "Bioterrorism Preparedness Program: Botulism and Bioterrorism," *Healthri*, 2. http://www.healthri.org/environment/biot/botulism.htm. See also, Stephen S. Arnon, Robert Schechter, Thomas V. Inglesby, et al., "Botulinum Toxin as a Biological Weapon: Medical and Public Health Issues, JAMA, February 28, 2001, 285 (8). Available on http://jama.ama-assn.org/issues/v285n8/ffull/jst00017.html.

24. Luba Vangelova, "Botulinum Toxin: A Poison That Can Heal," FDA Web site, 2. http://www.fda.gov/fdac/095_bot.html.

25. Ibid., 1.

26. Ibid., 3.

27. Alan Rockoff, "Botox, Smoothing Out the Wrinkles," Medicine Net.com, 1. At http://www.focusonskin.com.

28. "Facts about Pneumonic Plague, " *CDC Website*, 1. At http://www.bt.cdc.gov/DocumentsApp/FactSheet/Plague/About.asp. Also of interest, Thomas V. Inglesby, David T. Dennis, Donald A. Henderson, et al., "Plague as a Biological Weapon: Medical and Public Health Issues, *JAMA*, May 3, 2000, 283 (17). Available on http://jama.ama-assn.org/issues/v283n17/ffull/jst90013.html.

29. For this and the immediately following quotes, see, David T. Dennis and James M. Hughes, "Multidrug Resistance in Plague," *The New England Journal of Medicine*, September 4, 1997, 337 (10), 337.

30. Dennis, 338. A full report of the case appears in Marc Galimand, Annie Guiyoule, Guy Gerbaud, et al., "Multidrug Resistance in *Yersinia pestis* Mediated by a Transferable Plasmid, *The New England Journal of Medicine*, September 4, 1997, 337 (10), 677-681.

31. Donald A. Henderson, Thomas V. Inglesby, John T. Bartlett, et al., "Smallpox as a Biological Weapon: Medical and Public Health Issues," *JAMA*, June 9, 1999, 281 (22), 4. Available on http://jama.ama-assn.org/issues/v281n22/ffull/jst90000. html.

32. Shannon Brownlee, "Everything You Ever Wanted to Know About Smallpox Bioterrorism, *Optimal Wellness Center* Web site, 2. At http://www.mercola.com /2001/nov/14/smallpox.htm.

33. Ibid., 1.

34. Quoted in ibid., 1.

35. Katherine A. Feldman, Russell E. Enscore, Sarah L. Lathrop, et al., "An Outbreak of Primary Pneumonic Tularemia on Martha's Vineyard," *The New England Journal of Medicine*, November 29, 2001, 345 (22), 1602.

36. Danette L. Sutton, "Tularemia as A Biological Weapon," *Caduceus Institute of Classical Homeopathy* Web site, 1. At http://www.homeopathyhome.com/ caduceus/bioweapons2.html.

37. David T. Dennis, Thomas V. Inglesby, Donald A. Henderson, et al., "Tularemia as a Biological Weapon: Medical and Public Health Management," *JAMA*, June 6, 2001, 285 (21), 3. Available on http://jama.ama-assn.org/issues/v285n21/ffull/ jst10001.html.

38. Feldman, 1601.

39. Dennis, 8.

40. For details, see Laurie Garrett, *The Coming Plague: Newly Emerging Diseases* (New York: Farrar, Straus and Giroux, 1994), 73–83.

41. Ibid., 91–92.

42. Ibid., 28.

43. Ibid., 17, 27–28.

44. Ibid., 27.

45. "Crimean-Congo Haemorrhagic Fever," WHO Fact Sheets No. 208, 1. *WHO* Web site. At http://www.who.int/inf-fs/en/fact208.html.

46. Bob Swanepoel, "Congo Fever, some fascinating facts, 1. Found at http://www. uct.ac.za/depts/mmi/stannard/bog.html.

47. Ibid., 2.

48. James H.S. Gear, "Congo-Crimean Haemorrhagic Fever," *SAMJ*, October 1982, 62, 576.

49. S. P. Fisher-Hoch, J.A. Khan, S. Rehman, et al, "Crimean Congo-haemorrhagic fever treated with oral ribavirin," *Lancet*, August 19, 1995, 346 (8973), 472–5.

50. Garrett, *Coming*, 539.

51. Ibid.

52. Ibid, 536.

53. "How is Hantavirus Transmitted? The Rodent Connection, *CDC Special Pathogens Branch* Web site, 1. Located at http://cdc.gov/ncidod/diseases/hanta/hps/ noframes/transmit.htm.

54. "What Is the Treatment for HPS?" *CDC Special Pathogens Branch* Web site, 1. Located at http://cdc.gov/ncidod/diseases/hanta/hps/noframes/transmit.htm.

55. These statistics come from John W. King and Anurag Markanday, "Ebola Virus," *eMedicine Journal*, January 31, 2002, 3 (1), 3. http://www.emedicine.com/med/ topics626.htm; and from WHO, *WHO recommended Guidelines for Epidemic Preparedness and Response: Ebola Haemorrhagic Fever*, 12.

56. Ibid., 2.
57. Ibid., 3.
58. Garrett, *Coming,* 123, 124.
59. King, 6.
60. Garrett, *Coming,* 53–59.
61. Ibid., 255.
62. Ibid., 258.
63. Ibid., 258.
64. Ibid., 257.
65. Disease Information: Brucellosis (*Brucella melitensis, abortus, suis, and acanis*), CDC Division of Bacterial and Mycotic Diseases, *CDC* Web site, 1. At http://www. cdc.gov/ncidod/dbmd/diseaseinfo/brucellosis_t.htm.
66. Seymour M. Hersh, *Chemical and Biological Warfare: America's Hidden Arsenal* (Garden City, NY: Anchor Books, 1969), 74.
67. Ibid., 67.
68. FDA, Center for Food Safety and Applied Nutrition, "*Clostridium perfringens,*" in *Bad Bug Book* Web site, 2. At http://vm.cfsan.fda.gov/~mow/chp11.html
69. Ibid., 2.
70. Ibid., 3.
71. Eric Schlosser, *Fast Food Nation: The Dark Side of the All-American Meal* (Boston: Houghton Mifflin, 2001), 195.
72. Ibid., 195.
73. "Special Weapons Primer," *Federation of American Scientists* Web site, 4. At http://www.fas.org/nuke/intro/bw/agent.htm.
74. "Glanders," Field Manual, *NBC Med* Web site, 1. At http://www.nbc-med.org/ SiteConent/MedRef/OnlineRef/FieldManuals/medman/Glanders.htm.
75. Ibid., 1.
76. Ibid., 2.
77. Arjun Srinivasan, Carl N. Kraus, David DeShazer, et al., "Glanders in a Military Research Biologist," *The New England Journal of Medicine,* July 26, 2001, 345 (4), 258.
78. Ibid., 259.
79. Ibid., 259.
80. "Q Fever," Field Manual, *NBC Med* Web site, 1. At http://www.nbc-med.org/Site-Conent/MedRef/OnlineRef/FieldManuals/medman/Qfever.htm.
81. Murphy, 41.
82. "Ricin," Field Manual, *NBC Med* Web site, 1. At http://www.nbc-med.org/Site-Conent/MedRef/OnlineRef/FieldManuals/medman/Ricin.htm.
83. FDA, Center for Food Safety and Applied Nutrition, "Staphylococcus enterotoxin type B," in *Bad Bug Book* Web site, 2. At http://vm.cfsan.fda.gov/~mow/chp11. html
84. FDA, "Staphylococcus enterotoxin type B," 2.
85. Schlosser, 206.
86. Ibid.
87. Ibid., 210.
88. Ibid., 211.
89. Ibid., 211–12.
90. Ibid., 212.

91. Miller, 56–57.

92. Garrett, *Coming*, 522.

93. See H.R. Nayer, "Tuberculosis," in *Collier's Encyclopedia* (New York: MacMillan Educational Company, 1981), Vol, 22, 503.

94. Garrett, *Coming*, 524.

95. Ibid., 524.

96. Ibid., 525.

97. Ibid., 522.

98. Ibid., 527.

99. Quoted in "Nipah Virus a Rare New Genus—Study," *Earthchanges* Web site, 2. At http://www.earthchangestv.com.

100. "Nipah Virus a Rare New Genus," 2.

101. "Update: Outbreak of Nipah Virus—Malaysia and Singapore, 1999," *MMWR*, May 28, 2000. *CDC* Web site, 1. At http://www.cdc.gov/mmwr/preview/mmwrhtml/00057012.htm.

102. "Nipah Virus Fact Sheet," *WHO Information* Web site, 2. At http://www.who.int/inf-fs/en/fact262.html.

103. "Tick Borne Encephalitis," *Ireleth* Web site, 1. At http://www.ireleth.demon.co.uk/infection/virus/tickencepth.htm.

104. "Outbreak of Powassan Encepthalitis—Maine and Vermont, 1999-2001," *MMWR*, October 24-31, 2001, 286 (16), 761. Available at http://jama.ama-assn.org//issues/v286n16/ffull/jwp1024-1.html.

105. "Outbreak of Powassan Encepthalitis," 763.

106. Charlotte A. Bassett, "Yellow Fever," *Collier's Encyclopedia* , Volume 23, 690.

107. Garrett, *Coming*, 68.

108. Ibid., 70.

109. Ibid., 68.

110. Lesley Doyal and Imogen Pennell, *The Political Economy of Health* (London: Pluto Press, 1979), 242.

111. Ibid., 243.

112. Ibid., 243.

113. Ibid., 244.

114. Ibid., 275.

115. Ibid., 108.

116. Ibid., 109.

117. Sally F. Griffith, "'A Total Dissolution of the Bonds of Society': Community Death and Regeneration in Matthew Carey's S*hort Account of the Malignant Fever*," in *A Melancholy Scene of Devastation: The Public Response to the 1793 Philadelphia Yellow Fever Epidemic*, J. Worth Estes and Billy G. Smith, editors (Philadelphia: Science History Publications, 1997), 48. In the last part of the passage Griffith is quoting Matthew Carey.

118. Ibid., 48.

119. Phillip Lapsansky, "Abagail, A Negress": The Role and Legacy of African Americans in the Yellow Fever Epidemic, in Estes and Smith, 63.

120. Martin S. Pernick, "Politics, Parties, and Pestilence: Epidemic Yellow Fever in Philadelphia and the Rise of First Party Politics," in Estes and Smith, 129.

121. Lapsansky, 63. In our second transtional sequence, by the way, we will have more to say about Rush's treatment.

122. Pernick, 130–36.
123. Ibid., 130–34.
124. Gary Null (with James Feast), *AIDS: A Second Opinion* (New York: Seven Stories, 2002), 292-293.
125. Hakim Bey, *T.A.Z.: The Temporary Autonomous Zone, Ontological Anarchy and Poetic Terrorism* (New York: Autonomedia, 1985), 98.
126. Jean Steinmann, *Pascal*, Martin Turnell, translator (New York: Harcourt, Brace, and World, 1965), 107-108.
127. Ibid., 108.

PART II: TRADITIONAL TREATMENTS

1. Erich Jantsch, *The Self-Organizing Universe: Scientific and Human Implications of the Emerging Paradigm of Evolution* (Oxford: Pergamon Press, 1980), 108.
2. William H. McNeill, *Plagues and People* (Garden City, NY: Anchor Books, 1976), 53.
3. Christopher Wills, *Yellow Fever, Black Goddess: The Coevolution of People and Plagues* (Reading: Mass.: Helix Books, 1996), 47.
4. McNeill, 103.
5. McNeill, 137-138.
6. Garth L. Nicolson, Meryl Nass, and Nancy L. Nicolson, "Anthrax Vaccine: Controversy Over Safety and Efficacy," *Antibiotics and Infectious Disease Newsletter* (np: Elsevier Science, 2000), 3. Available at http://www.enter.net/~jfsorg/Official-Documents_files/Nicoloson.htm.
7. Nicolson, 3.
8. Kevin Hoffman, "The Anthrax Vaccine: Read This Before You Take It," *Cleveland Free Times*, November 7-13, 2001, 5.
9. Ibid., 5.
10. Nicolson, 4.
11. Ibid., 3–4.
12. Ibid., 4.
13. Hoffman, 1.
14. Ibid.
15. Ibid., 2.
16. Ibid.
17. Ibid.
18. Ibid.
19. McNeill, 238.
20. AMNews staff, "Air Force physician faces court-martial over refusal to get anthrax vaccine," Amednews.com, January 29, 2001, 1. At http://www.ama-assn.org/sci-pubs/amnews/pick_01/hlsd0129.htm
21. "Court Martial in Anthrax Clash: Air Force Major Refuses Vaccine; Pentagon Insists Its Safe: Records: At Least 100 Service Members Got Sick," *Optimal Wellness* Web site, 1. At http://www.mercola.com/2000'feb/6/anthrax_clash.htm.
22. Ibid., 2.
23. Ibid., 2.
24. Julie Klotter, "Antthrax Vaccine," *Townsend Letter for Doctors and Patients*, January 2002, 1.
25. Ibid., 1.

26. John F. Modlin, Dixie E. Snider, Dennis A. Brooks, et al. "Use of Anthrax Vaccine in the United States: Recommendations of the Advisory Committee on Immunization Practices, *MMWR*, December 15, 2000, 49 (RR15), 9.

27. Ibid.

28. Hoffman, 5.

29. Nicolson, 2.

30. See Walene James, *Immunization: The Reality Behind the Myth* (Westport, Conn.: Bergin and Garvey, 1995), 9–10.

31. "Executive Summary [of the Rep. Jack Metcalf's House Study]," *DSNurse*, November, 11, 2001, 1. Available at http://home.att.net/~dstormmom/metcalf.htm.

32. Nicolson, 3.

33. Hoffman, 5.

34. Doctors for Disaster Preparedness, "Statement for the Record [for the March Hearings on the DoD's Anthrax Vaccine Program," *Doctors for Disaster Preparedness* Web site, 2. At http://www.oism.org/ddp/anthddp.htm.

35. Nicolson, 5.

36. Ibid.

37. Ibid., 4.

38. Julian Borger, "Anthrax Killer could grow more bacteria," *Guardian Weekly*, June 27–July 3, 2002, 4.

39. "Patient Information: Ciprofloxacin 500 mg, Oral Tablet" *CDC Public Health Emergency Preparedness and Awareness* Web site, 1. At http://www.bt.cdc.gov/DocumentsApp/Anthrax/10312001/cipro.asp.

40. Shankar Vedantam, "Prescribing Cipro Is 'Uncontrolled Experiment': Health Officials Worry That Taking Drug for Anthrax May Have Serious Side Effects," *Washington Post*, November 3, 2001, A15.

41. Vedantam, A15.

42. "Ciprofloxacin Use," *MMWR*, 2001.

43. "Cipro Can Be Harmful," *Holistic-online* Web site, 1. At http://holisticonline.com/Remedies/biot_anthrax-cipro-can-be-harmful.htm.

44. The Cohen article is reviewed in Vladimir S. Shoukhov, "New article on ciproflaxacin side effects," *e-drug* Web site, 2. At http://old.healthnet.org/programs/e-drug-hma/e-drug200111/ms00013.html.

45. As quoted in "Ciprofloxacin side effects ranged up to 19% in postal workers," *Center for Infectious Disease* Web site, 1. At http://www1.umn.edu./cidrap/content/bioprep.news/sideeffects113001.html.

46. "Patient Information: Ciprofloxacin," 1.

47. Thomas V. Inglesby, Donald A. Henderson, John G. Bartlett, et al., "Anthrax as Biological Weapon: Medical and Public Health Management," *JAMA*, May 12, 1999, 281 (18), 9. Available on http://jama.ama-assn.org/issues/v281n19/ffull/ jst800 27.html.

48. "Fact Sheet: Ciprofloxacin," *New Mexico AIDS Infonet* Web site, 1. At http://www.aidsinfonet.org/531-cipro.html.

49. Wills, 164.

50. Ibid., 165.

51. Bayer, "Cipro® (ciprofloxacin hydrochloride) tablets," 4. This material can be reached via the *FDA* Web site. See http://www.fda.gov/cder/foi/label/2000/20780S08lbl.pdf.

52. Wills, 251.

53. Vedantam, A15.

54. Ibid.

55. Ibid.

56. Ibid.

57. "Virazole Inhalation: Pharmacology and Chemistry," *Medscape Pharmacotherapy* Web site, 19. At http://www.medscape.com.

58. "Virazole Inhalation: Patient Handout," *Medscape DrugInfo* Web site, at http:// promini.medscape.com.

59. Ibid., 8.

60. Ibid.

61. Ibid., 9.

62. Ibid., 10.

63. Ibid.

64. Ibid., 11.

65. Ibid.

66. Infectious Diseases and Immunization Committee, Canadian Pediatric Society, "Ribavirin: Is there a risk to hospital personnel?" *Canadian Medical Association Journal*, 1991, 144 (3), 285.

67. California Department of Health Services, "Hazard Alert: Ribavirin," California Governor's Homepage, 2. At http://www.dhs.cahwnet.gov/HESIS/riba.htm.

68. James, 37.

69. See Peter Sloterdijk, *Critique of Cynical Reason*, trans. Michael Eldred (Minneapolis: University of Minnesota Press, 1987).

70. Margaret O. Hyde and Elizabeth H. Forsyth, *Vaccinations: From Smallpox to Cancer* (New York: Franklin Watts, 2000), 33.

71. Hyde, 33–34.

72. Nerissa Pacio, "Trials of 50-Year-Old Smallpox Vaccine Underway in U.S.; Bioterrorism: Volunteers receive diluted versions to gauge the side effects and its effectiveness," *Los Angeles Times,* July 9, 2002, 15.

73. Pacio, 15.

74. "Mass smallpox vaccination can cut deaths," *UPI,* July 9, 2002.

75. Ibid.

76. Ibid.

77. "Smallpox: CDC advisers lobby for 'ring containment' smallpox vaccine," *Medical Letter on the CDC & FDA,* July 7, 2002, NewsRx.com and NewsRx.net, 13.

78. Keith Bradsher, "The Treatments: 3 Small Companies Say Their Vaccines Are Cheaper," *New York Times*, November 8, 2001.

79. Richard Wenzel, "Exposure Danger Too Great for Vaccination to be Voluntary," *Richmond Times-Dispatch,* July 10, 2002, A-11.

80. Lawrence K. Altman, "Smallpox Proposal Raises Ethical Issues," *The New York Times,* June 22, 2002, A9.

81. Altman, A9.

82. Susan Okie, "U.S. Officials Want A Dose for Every Person in the Country by the End of 2002, *Washington Post*, October 28, 2001, A-18.

83. Okie, A-18.

84. "Smallpox Vaccine: Panel's Recommendation Raises Concern," *American Health Line,* June 25, 2002.

85. Altman, A9.
86. "Smallpox: Doctors poorly informed about side effects of vaccine, survey finds, " *Medical Letter on the CDC & FDA* , June 29, 2002, NewsRx.com and NewsRx.net.
87. "Smallpox Vaccine: Doctors and the Public Lack Knowledge," American Health Line, May 10, 2002.
88. Tina Hesman, "Forum Reflects Controversy Over Smallpox Vaccine; Views Range From 'Over My Dead Body' to Making It Available to Everyone," *St. Louis Post-Dispatch* , June 9, 2002, C2.
89. Gro Harlem Brundtland, "Statement to the Press by the Director-General of the World Health Organization, *WHO* Web site, 1. At http://www.who.int/inf-pr-2001/en/state2001-16.html.
90. Okie, A-18.
91. Ibid.
92. Bradsher.
93. James Odell, "Vaccines—What's in the Next Cauldron?" *Townsend Letter for Doctors and Patients*, January 2002, 114.
94. Odell, 114, citing the February 1994 issue of *Scientific American*.
95. Ibid.
96. Ibid.
97. Ibid.
98. Gary Null (with James Feast), *AIDS: A Second Opinion* (New York: Seven Stories, 2002), 391–99.
99. Odell, 114.
100. Donald A. Henderson and Bernard Moss, *Vaccines* (Washington, D.C.: NIH), Chapter 6, 1.
101. Hyde, 10.
102. Ibid.
103. Henderson, Chapter 6, 3.
104. Ibid.
105. Gary Null, *Vaccines: A Second Opinion*, unpublished ms., 159.
106. Miller, cited in Null, *Vaccines,* 161.
107. Henderson, Chapter 6, 4.
108. Hyde, 15.
109. Thomas McKeown, *The Modern Rise of Population* (New York: Academic Press, 1976), 68.
110. McKeown, 12–13.
111. Ibid., 78.
112. Ibid., 79.
113. McNeill, 45.
114. Quoted in McKeown, 75.
115. McNeill, 198.
116. Ibid., 199.
117. Ibid., 96.
118. Ibid., 93.
119. Ibid., 142.
120. Ibid., 135.
121. Ibid., 137.
122. Quoted in McKeown, 135.

123. Quoted in McKeown,136.

124. McKeown, 162, his emphasis.

125. Quoted in Philip Incao, "Incao's Hepatitis B Vaccination Testimony in Ohio," March 1, 1999, 3. Available at garynull.com.

126. Incao, 2.

127. Harold E. Buttram, "Vaccine Scene 2001: Update and Overview," 3. Available on GaryNull.com.

128. Hyde, 64.

129. Ibid.

130. James, 9.

131. Hyde, 59–60.

132. Australian Vaccination Network, *Vaccination Roulette: Experiences, risks, and alternatives* (Bangalow, Australia: AVN, 1998), 101.

133. Ibid.,101.

134. Gary Null, *Get Healthy Now* (New York: Seven Stories, 1999), 841.

135. Vaccine Injury Alliance, "Vaccine Related Injuries," 2, *Vaccine Injury Alliance* Web site. At http://www.vaccineinjury.org.

136. James, 9.

137. Hyde, 60.

138. Harold W. Clark, "Mycoplasma Contaminated Vaccines, *Townsend Letter for Doctors and Patients*, January 2002, 110.

139. Ibid.

140. Ibid.

141. Ibid.

142. T. Curtis, "The Origin of AIDS," *Rolling Stone*, March 19, 1992, 54.

143. Ibid.

144. "Safety, Efficacy, Heart of Vaccine Use: Experts Discuss Pros, Cons,"*DVM*, December 1986, 18. The entire passage is found in Null, *AIDS,* 308.

145. Curtis, 54.

146. Ibid.

147. Ibid. The entire passage is from Null, *AIDS,* 312.

148. Ibid. Null, *AIDS,* 313.

149. Ibid.

150. Ibid. Null, *AIDS,* 313.

151. Cited in Incao, 3.

152. Incao, 3.

153. Buttram, 3.

154. Ibid.

155. Quoted in Buttram, 4.

156. Buttram, 3.

157. Ibid.

158. Ibid.

159. Ibid., 5.

160. Ibid., 5.

161. Incao, 3.

162. Australian Vaccination Network, 24.

163. Cited in James, 12.

164. Ibid.

165. Australian Vaccination Network, 24.
166. Ibid., 25.
167. Ibid., 24.
168. Buttram, 2–3.
169. Ibid., 4.
170. Tom Bethel, "Shots in the Dark, *American Spectator*, 1999, 2. Available on garynull.com.
171. Ibid.
172. Hyde, 38.
173. Ibid.
174. Bethel, 1.
175. Incao, 2.
176. Buttram, 2.
177. Bethel, 2.
178. Ibid.
179. Ibid., 1.
180. Ibid.
181. Australian Vaccination Network, 12.
182. Buttram, 7.
183. Ibid.
184. Australian Vaccination Network, 12.
185. James, 16, quoting from Richard Moskowitz, "The Case Against Immunization," *American Journal of Homeopathy*, 76 (March 1983).
186. Quoted in *Australian Vaccination Network*, 11.
187. Cited in James, 16.
188. Philip F. Incao, "How Vaccination Works: Will this unorthodox view gain serious consideration?" *The Natural Immunity Network.*, 2. Available on garynull.com.
189. Buttram, 5.
190. Australian Vaccination Network, 13.
191. James, 14.
192. Buttram, 5.
193. Incao, "How Vaccination Works," 3.
194. Ibid.
195. Bruno Bettelheim, *The Uses of Enchantment: The Meaning and Importance of Fairy Tales* (New York: Vintage Books, 1975), 7.
196. Hyde, 50.
197. Quoting Michael Verney-Elliot, "AIDS Vaccines—The Cruel Delusion," *Continuum*, 5 (2): 7 (Winter 1997/1998), 6.; in Null, *AIDS*, 397.
198. Null, "Vaccines," 162.
199. Continuing the same Verney-Elliot quote, in Null, *AIDS*, 397.
200. James, 182.
201. Ibid., 178.
202. Ibid., 163.
203. Ibid., 182.
204. Ibid., 181.
205. Ibid., 150.
206. Australian Vaccination Network, 9.

207. Ibid., 10.

208. Incao, "How Vaccination Works," 3.

209. Sara E. Melzer, *Discourses of the Fall: A Study of Pascal's* Pensées (Berkeley: University of California Press, 1986), 95.

210. Quoted in Ernest Mortimer, *Blaise Pascal: Life and Work of a Realist* (London: Methuen and Co., 1959), 190.

211. Melzer, 104.

212. Blaise Pascal, *Pensées*, H. F. Stewart, translator (New York: Pantheon Books, 1950), 101.

213. Melzer, 105.

214. Blaise Pascal, *The Provincial Letters*, M. J. Krailsheimer, translator (London, Penguin Books, 1967), 99. The book was originally published in 1656.

215. Ibid., 99.

216. Ibid., 82.

217. Ibid., 83

218. Ibid., 104.

219. Ibid., 104, 108.

220. Thomas Kuhn, *The Structure of Scientific Revolutions* (Chicago: University of Chicago Press, 1970).

221. John Harvey Powell, *Bring Out Your Dead: The Great Plague of Yellow Fever in Philadelphia in 1793* (New York: Arno Press, 1970), 78. This is a reprint of the 1949 edition.

222. Ibid., 80.

223. Ibid., 81.

224. Ibid., 42.

225. Ibid., 172, 173.

226. Ibid., 169.

227. Ibid., 121, 122.

228. Ibid., 301.

229. Ibid., 131–32.

PART III: NATURAL WAYS TO WARD OFF THE INCURSION OF NEW GERMS

1. Stephen E. Straus, "Comprehensive Medical Care for Bioterrorism Exposure: Are We Making Evidence-Based Decisions?: Testimony Before the House Committee on Government Reform," *NCCAM* Web site, 2. At http://nccam.nih.gov/ne/testimony/bio-full.htm.

2. Garth Nicolson, "Dietary Considerations for Patients with Chronic Illnesses and Multiple Chronic Infections: A Brief Outline of Eighteen Dietary Steps to Better Health," *Townsend Letter for Doctors and Patients*, October 2001. Can be located at http://www.findarticles.com/cf_0/m0ISW/2001_Oct/78900838/print.jhtml.

3. Nicolson, 2.

4. Ibid., 3.

5. Ibid.

6. Leo Galland, "Eating Safely in a Polluted World: Part I—You Don't Have to Choose Between Microbes and Chemicals," *HealthWorld* Web site, 2. At http://www.healthy.net.

7. Majid Ali, "The Seventh Path: Optimal Hydration, and Nutrient and Herbal Support of Body Ecosystems," *Aging Healthy Virtual Library*, 1. At http://www.majidali.com/Vol%201%20No%202%20%20The%Seventh%Path.htm.
8. Galland, 2.
9. Ibid., 4.
10. Mark Harris, "The Benefits of Meditation: Healing Through Feeling and Awareness," *Conscious Choice* Web site, 3. At http://www.consciouschoice.com/health/meditation1103.html.
11. Ibid., 4.
12. Pichichero, M. E., et al., "Outcomes after Judicious Antibiotic Use for Respiratory Tract Infections Seen in a Private Pediatric Practice," *Pediatrics*, April 2000,105 (4): 753–59.
13. "Consuming Chinese Herbs May Cause Kidney Failure." *AORN Journal* online, April 2000, 1.
14. Rob McCaleb, "JAMA bashes herbs for surgical patients, Herb Research Foundation News, *Herb World News Online* Web site, 1. At http://herbs.org/current/jama.htm.
15. Cindy Brumley, "Herbs and the Perioperative Patient," *AORN Journal* online, November 2000, 4.
16. Ibid., 2.
17. Kerry Bone, "Safety Issues in Herbal Medicine: Adulteration, Adverse Reactions and Organ Toxicities," *Townsend Letter for Doctors and Patients* online, October 2001, 2.
18. James A. Duke, "Death by Pharmaceuticals? (health risks of herbal dietary supplements)," *Better Nutrition* online, June 2001, 1.
19. Jack Challem, "The Problem With Herbs," *Natural Health* online, January 1999, 1.
20. Ibid., 3.
21. Challem, 3.
22. Judy Krizmanic, "How fresh are your herbs? Using your senses can help you find quality specimens," *Vegetarian Times* online Web site, January 1996, 2, 3.
23. Kathi Keville, "Herbs that love your liver: enhance the health of this vital organ," *Vegetarian Times* online, August 1996, 3.
24. L. C. Mishra, et al., "Scientific basis for the therapeutic use of Withania somnifera (*ashwagandha*): a review," *Alternative Medicine Review*, August 2000, 5 (4): 334–46.
25. L. Davis, et al., "Immunomodulatory activity of *Withania somnifera*," *Journal of Ethnopharmacology*, July 2000, 71 (1-2):193-200; and J. Dhuley, "Therapeutic efficacy of Ashwagandha against experimental aspergillosis in mice" *Immunopharmacology and Immunotoxicology*, February1998, 20 (1):191–8.
26. Janet Zand, "On Echinacea and Goldenseal," *HealthWorld* online Web site, 1. At http://www.healthy.net.
27. See Z. Zakay-Rones, et al. "Inhibition of several strains of influenza virus in vitro and reduction of symptoms by an elderberry extract (*Sambucus nigra L.*) during an outbreak of influenza B Panama," *Journal of Alternative and Complementary Medcine*, Winter 1995, 1(4): 361–9.
28. Delaha et al., "Inhibition of mycobacteria by garlic extract (*Allium sativum*)," *Antimicrobial Agents and Chemotherapy*, April 1985, 27 (4):485-6; and L. Davis et al., "In vitro synergism of concentrated *Allium sativum* extract and *amphotericin.B* against *Cryptococcus neoformans*.," *Planta Medica*, December 1994, 60 (6): 546–9.

29. N. L. Guo, et al. "Demonstration of the anti-viral activity of garlic extract against human cytomegalovirus in vitro," *Chinese Medical Journal (English)*, February 1993, 106 (2): 93–6; N. D. Weber, et al., "In vitro viricidal effects of *Allium sativum* (garlic) extract and compounds," *Planta Medica*, October 1992, 58 (5): 417–23; A.V. Tatarintsev, et al., "The ajoene blockade of integrin-dependent processes in an HIV-infected cell system. [Russian]," *Vestn Ross Akad Med Nauk*, 1992 (11–12): 6–10; and B. Foster, et al., "An in vitro evaluation of human cytochrome p450 3a4 and p-glycoprotein inhibition by garlic," *Journal of Pharmaceutical Pharmacology Science*, May–August 2001, 4(2): 176–84.

30. David L. Hoffman, "Garlic," *HealthWorld* online Web site, 1 at http://www.healthy.net.

31. "Antimicrobial Agents and Chemotherpeutic Effects of Garlic Clarified," *Doctor's Guide: Personal Edition* Web site, 1. At http://www.docguide.com.

32. "Antimicrobial Agents and Chemotherpeutic Effects of Garlic," 1.

33. Joseph Mercola, "Raw Garlic for Parasites and Viral Infections," *Optimal Wellness Center* Web site, 4. At http://www.mercola.com/2001/mar/garlic_infections.htm.

34. Douglas Dupler, "American Ginseng," *Gale Encyclopedia of Alternative Medicine* Web site, 2.

35. M. Davydov, et al., "*Eleutherococcus senticosus* (Rupr. & Maxim.) Maxim. (*Araliaceae*) as an adaptogen: a closer look." *Journal of Ethnopharmacology*, October 2000, 72 (3): 345–93.

36. Brumley, 7.

37. Zand, 1.

38. T. S. Yam, et al., "Microbiological activity of whole and fractionated crude extracts of tea (*Camellia sinensis*), and of tea components," *FEMS Microbiology Letter*, July 1, 1997, 152 (1):69–74; M. Shetty, et al., "Antibacterial activity of tea (*Camellia sinensis*) and coffee (*Coffee arabica*) with special reference to *Salmonella typhimurium*," *Journal of Communicable Disease*, September1994, 26 (3): 147–50; Y. Okai, et al., "Potent suppressing activity of the non-polyphenolic fraction of green tea (*Camellia sinensis*) against genotoxin-induced umu C gene expression in *Salmonella typhimurium* (TA 1535/pSK 1002)—association with pheophytins a and b," *Terato Carcinog Mutagen*, 1997–98,17 (6): 305–12; H. Chosa, et al., "Antimicrobial and microbicidal activities of tea and catechins against Mycoplasm," *Kansenshogaku Zasshi*, May 1992, 66 (5): 606–11. (Japanese); and M. Toda, et al. "Antibacterial and bactericidal activities of Japanese green tea," *Nippon Saikingaku Zasshi*, July 1989, 44 (4): 669–72. (Japanese).

39. Sugita-Konishi Y, et al., "Epigallocatechin gallate and gallocatechin gallate in green tea catechins inhibit extracellular release of Vero toxin from enterohemorrhagic *Escherichia coli* O157:H7," *Biochim Biophys Acta*, October 18, 1999, 1472 (1-2): 42–50.

40. T. S. Yam, et al., "The effect of a component of tea (*Camellia sinensis*) on methicillin resistance, PBP2' synthesis, and beta-lactamase production in *Staphylococcus aureus*," *J Antimicrob Chemother*, August 1998, 42 (2): 211–6; and J.M. Hamilton-Miller, et al., "Disorganization of cell division of methicillin-resistant *Staphylococcus aureus* by a component of tea (*Camellia sinensis*): a study by electron microscopy. *FEMS Microbiology Letter*, July 15, 1999,176 (2): 463–9.

41. S. P. Pillai, et al., "The ability of certain antimutagenic agents to prevent development of antibiotic resistance," *Mutat Res*, September 20, 2001, 496 (1–2): 61–73.

42. Y. Sun, et al., "Immune restoration and/or augmentation of local graft versus host reaction by traditional Chinese medicinal herbs," *Cancer,* July 1,1983, 52 (1): 70–73; Y. Sun, et al., "Preliminary observations on the effects of the Chinese medicinal herbs *Astragalus membranaceus* and *Ligustrum lucidum* on lymphocyte blastogenic responses, *J Biol Response Mod* , 1983, 2 (3): 227–37; Yim, et al., "Hepatoprotective action of an oleanolic acid-enriched extract of *Ligustrum lucidum* fruits is mediated through an enhancement on hepatic glutathione regeneration capacity in mice," *Phytother Res,* November 15, 2001,15 (7): 589–92; and B. H. Lau, et al., "Chinese medicinal herbs inhibit growth of murine renal cell carcinoma," *Cancer Biother,* Summer 1994, 9 (2): 153–61.
43. Keville, 2.
44. Penny King, "12 herbs that experts couldn't live without," *Vegetarian Times* online Web site, September 1997, 3.
45. David L. Hoffmann, "Myrrh," *Herbal Materai Medica* Web site, 2.
46. Mark Mayell, "Maitake Extracts and Their Therapeutic Potential—A Review," *Alternative Medicine Review* Web site, February 2001, 1.
47. Ibid., 9.
48. S. Sarkar, et al., "Antiviral effect of the extract of culture medium of *Lentinus edodes mycelia* on the replication of herpes simplex virus type 1," *Antiviral Res* , April 1993, 20 (4): 293–303; and H. Suzuki, et al., "Inhibition of the infectivity and cytopathic effect of human immunodeficiency virus by water-soluble lignin in an extract of the culture medium of *Lentinus edodes mycelia* (LEM)," April 14, 1989, 160 (1): 367–73.
49. Y. Yamamoto, et al., "Immunopotentiating activity of the water-soluble lignin rich fraction prepared from LEM—the extract of the solid culture medium of *Lentinus edodes mycelia,*" *Biosci Biotechnol Biochem* , November 1997, 61 (11): 1909–12.
50. S. Y. Wang, et al., "The anti-tumor effect of *Ganoderma lucidum* is mediated by cytokines released from activated macrophages and T lymphocytes," *International Journal of Cancer,* March 17, 1997, 70 (6): 699–705; S. K. Eo, et al., "Antiviral activities of various water and methanol soluble substances isolated from *Ganoderma lucidum,*" Journal of Ethnopharmacology, December 15, 1999, 68 (1–3): 129–36; and B. S. Min, et al., "Triterpenes from the spores of *Ganoderma lucidum* and their inhibitory activity against HIV-1 protease," *Chem Pharm Bull* (Tokyo), October 1998, 46 (10): 1607–12.
51. "The Olive Leaf—A Rising Herbal Star Healing Infections and Much, Much More," *Health/Science Newsletter* Web site, 1997, 1. At http://www.asktom-naturally.com/naturally/hsnltr.html.
52. Ibid., 2.
53. Quoted in ibid., 3. See also, "Morton Walker, "Olive Leaf Extract as a Main Therapy in the Antimicrobial Supermarket," *Townsend Letter for Doctors and Patients,* May 2001.
54. Both quotes from Gregory S. Kelly, "Rhodiola rosea: A Possible Plant Adaptogen (evaluation of therapeutic properties," *Alternative Medicine Review,* June 2001, 2.
55. Belinda Rowland, "Schisandra," *Gale Encyclopedia of Alternative Medicine* Web site, 1.
56. David Hoffmann, *The Herbal Handbook: A User's Guide to Medical Herbalism* (Rochester, Vermont: Healing Arts Press, 1987), 36.

57. Victoria Stagg Elliott, "Depression, anxiety still common complaints after Sept. 11: A war, terrorism, and the sluggish economy have left many at-risk patients struggling to cope," *Amednews.com* , January 7, 2002, 1. At http://www.ama-assn. org/sci-pubs/anmnews/pick_02/hlsd0107.htm.

58. Ibid., 1.

59. Majid Ali, "Nutrient and Herbal Support for Stress, *Aging Healthy Virtual Library*, 1. At http://www.majidali.com/Vol%201%202No%20Nutrients%for%stress.htm.

60. "Supplement to: The Art of Getting Well, Bee Pollen: The Perfect Food," Arthritis Trust of America Web site, 1. At www.arthritistrust.com.

61. Ibid., 2.

62. Ibid., 7.

63. Ibid., 9.

64. Brenda Adderly, "The Latest Buzz on Products of the Hive, *Better Nutrition* Web site, August 1999, 1.

65. Ibid., 3.

66. "Science News, Propolis heals herpes lesions faster than acyclovir," *Herb World News online* Web site, 1. At http://www.herbs.org/current/propolis.htm.

67. "Supplement to: The Art of Getting Well, Bee Pollen," 10.

68. R. M. Loria and P. N. Huynh, "Regulation of the Immune Response by dehydroepiandrosterone and its metabolites," *Journal of Endocrinology*, 1996, 150: 0150–S209.

69. Julie A. McLachlan, Carla D. Serkin, and Ouahid Bakouche, "Dehydroepiandrosterone Modulation of Lipopolysaccharide-Stimulated Monocyte Cytotoxicity," *Journal of Immunology*, 1996.

70. "The Biology of Lactoferrin," *Confidential*, State Academy of Medicine, Tamaulipas, Mexico, 3. See also, Koji Nishiya and David A. Horowitz, "Contrasting Effects of Lactoferrin on Human Lymphocyte and Monocyte Natural Killer Activity and Antibody-Dependent Cell-Mediated Cytotoxicity," *Journal of Immunology*, 1982, 129 (6): 2519–23.

71. See "Nutrient highlights: Antioxidants," *garynull.com* Web site, 12. At http:// garynull.com/Documents/NutrientHighlights/AntiOx/Antioxidants.htm

72. Ibid., 1.

73. Karl Folkers, Manabu Morita, and Judson McRee, Jr., "The Activities of Coenzyme Q_{10} and Vitamin B_6 for Immune Response," *Biochemical and Biophysical Research Communications*, May 28, 1993, 193 (1): 88–92.

74. Gary Null, "The Antioxidant Vitamin: Vitamin C," *Townsend Letter for Doctors and Patients*, February/March 1994. 3. Available at http://garynull.com/Documents/vitaminc.htm.

75. Noted in Gary Null, "The Antioxidant Vitamin," 4.

76. Gary Null, "The Antioxidant Vitamin," 4.

77. Gary Null, "The Antioxidant Vitamin," 10. See also, R. Jacob, et al., "Immunocompetence and oxidant defense during ascorbate depletion of healthy men," *American Journal of Clinical Nutrition*, 1991, 54: 1302S–9S.

78. B. P. Yu, et al., "Can antioxidant supplementation slow the aging process?" *Biofactors*, 1998, 7, 93.

79. C. Fortes, et al., "The Effect of Zinc and Vitamin A Supplementation on Immune Response in an Older Population," *JAGS*, 1998, 46, 24.

80. E. Mocchegian et al., "Zinc and Immunoresistance to infection in aging: new biological tools," *TiPS*, June 2000, 21, 205.

81. See, L. Rink and H. Kirchner, "Zinc-Altered Immune Function and Cytokine Production," *Zinc and Health: Current Status and Future Directions*, 2000 Supplement, 1407S–1411S; M. Scott and K. Koski, "Zinc Deficiency Impairs Immune Response against Parasitic Nematode Infections at Intestinal and Systemic Sites," *Zinc and Health: Current Status and Future Directions*, 2000 Supplement, 1412S–1420S; M. Baum, G. Shor-Posner, and A. Campa, "Zinc Status in Human Immunodeficiency Virus Infection," *Zinc and Health: Current Status and Future Directions*, 2000 Supplement, 1421S–1423S; and S. Powell, "The Antioxidant Properties of Zinc," *Zinc and Health: Current Status and Future Directions*, 2000 Supplement, 1447S–1454S.

82. Michael Reed Gach, "What is Acupressure?" excerpt from *Acupressure's Potent Points*," from the Acupressure Institute, 3. See Web site at www.acupressure.com.

83. Gach, 3.

84. Ibid., 1.

85. Ibid.

86. Cited in "Biofeedback Indicates Drumming Relieves Stress," All One Tribe Foundation, 1. Available at http://www.awarenessmag.com/so7_bio.htm.

87. Barry Bittman, "Deep Within: Drumming as a Healing Strategy," *Mind-Body* Web site, 1. Available at http://www.mind-body.org/bittman%20%20deep%20within.htm.

88. Bittman, 1.

89. Todd A. Hoover, "Homeopathic Prophylaxis: Fact or Fiction," *National Center for Homeopathy* Web site, 1. At http://www.homeopathic.org/crtoddh.htm.

90. Ibid.

91. Ibid., 2.

92. Ibid.

93. Ibid., 5.

94. Ibid., 3.

95. Ibid., 5.

96. Julian Winston, "Historical Perspective, " *National Center for Homeopathy* Web site, 1. At http://www.homeopathic.org/crtoddh.htm.

97. Susan Curtis, *A Handbook of Homeopathic Alternatives to Immunization* (West Wickham, England: Winter Press, 1994), 8.

98. Ibid., 8.

99. Ibid., 9.

100. "Post Traumatic Disorder, Anxiety, Biological Attack," *National Center for Homeopathy* Web site, 3. At http://www.homeopathic.org/crattack.htm.

101. Thomas Levy, "Bioterrorism: Beyond Vaccinations and Antibiotics," *Opimal Wellness Center* Web site, 1. At http://www.mercola.com/2001/nov/17/bioterrorism.htm.

102. Ibid.

103. Ibid., 2.

104. "Natural Herbal Remedies for Anthrax: Echinacea," *Holisticonline* Web site, 1. At http://holisticonline.com/Remedies/Biot/biot_anthrax-echinacea-2_herb-rem.htm.

105. "Natural Herbal Remedies for Anthrax: Garlic," *Holisticonline* Web site, 1. At http://holisticonline.com/Remedies/Biot/biot_anthrax-natural-rem-garlic. htm.
106. "Natural Herbal Remedies for Anthrax: Vitamin A," *Holisticonline* Web site, 1. At http://holisticonline.com/Remedies/Biot/biot_anthrax-Vit-A-1-natural-rem. htm.
107. "Natural Herbal Remedies for Anthrax: Beta-Carotene and Immunity," *Holistic-online* Web site, 1. At http://holisticonline.com/Remedies/Biot/biot_anthrax-beta- car-2-nat-rem.htm.
108. Levy, 1.
109. "Homeopathic Remedies for Anthrax," *Holisticonline* Web site, 1. At http://holisticonline.com/Remedies/Biot/biot_anthrax-homeo-remedies-for-1.htm.

CONCLUSION

1. George H. Mead, *Mind, Self and Society from the Standpoint of a Social Behaviorist,* Charles W. Morris, editor (Chicago: University of Chicago Press, 1934), 343.
2. Ibid., 43.
3. Ibid., 171.
4. Blaise Pascal, *Pensées,* H. F. Stewart, translator (New York: Pantheon Books, 1950), 46–47.
5. Ibid., 69.
6. Ibid., 63.
7. Ernest Mortimer, *Blaise Pascal: Life and Work of a Realist* (London: Methuen and Co., 1959), 176.
8. Mathew Carey, *A Short Account of the Malignant Fever, Lately Prevalent in Philadelpia* (New York: Arno Press, 1970), 92. This is a reprint of the edition of January 16, 1794. Note, I have regularized the spelling.
9. Ibid., 25.
10. Ibid., 91.

CODA

1. Richard Preston, *The Cobra Event* (New York: Ballantine, 1997), 229.
2. Preston, 190–91.
3. Steve Dalachinsky, "the phone call (first time)," in *Morir Soñando: Poems of 9/11, etc.* (JVC Books: Arcadia, Fla., 2002), 15–16. This particular poem was written on October 5 and 6, 2001. Quoted with permission.

Index